"Reading *Teaching from the Heart* was a delight superseded only by getting to know Ms. Raper personally. She is an experienced and self-reflective teacher, and these qualities echo throughout her book. There are countless books in the marketplace about practicing and teaching yoga. It is refreshing therefore to read a book that elucidates the foundational aspects shaping the art and profession of yoga teaching. Read this book not only to educate yourself but also to feed your growth as a teacher and a person."

**– Judith Hanson Lasater, PT, Ph.D**
Yoga teacher since 1972 and author of 11 books, including the latest *Teaching Yoga with Intention*

"Sandy has thoughtfully curated a collection of lessons that covers so many important and often overlooked aspects of being a sustainable & impactful yoga teacher. Teaching yoga in our modern world has so many layers and can easily leave many teachers overwhelmed & burned out over time but this easy-to-read book provides the support and inspiration for teachers looking to be more potent in their teaching and more purposeful in their lives. An excellent resource for yoga teacher training programs to use to support their programs."

**– Tiffany Cruikshank, L.Ac., MAOM**
Founder of Yoga Medicine

"*Teaching from the Heart: Lessons on Developing Character, Confidence, and Leadership as a Yoga Teacher* by Sandy Raper offers a profound exploration of the deeper qualities that define a yoga teacher beyond the technical aspects of the practice.

Raper's personal journey, shared in the introduction, sets the tone for an inspiring and insightful read. With chapters dedicated to character development and the exploration of one's motivation and intention, this book provides aspiring, new, and seasoned yoga teachers with invaluable guidance and reflective exercises. Raper's emphasis on service and connection as the core of teaching resonates throughout, making it an indispensable resource for anyone seeking to teach yoga from the heart."

**– Stephanie Spence**

Yoga scholar and teacher, practitioner, and award-winning author of *Yoga Wisdom: Warrior Tales Inspiring You On And Off Your Mat*

# Teaching
## from the
# Heart

Lessons on Developing Character,
Confidence, and Leadership as a Yoga Teacher

SANDY RAPER

Foreword by Rolf Gates

ISBN: 979-8-9902839-0-9

# Teaching from the Heart

*In love and memory of my mom, Iris*

# Contents

# Foreword

When I first met Sandy Raper fifteen years ago, she was already an extremely respected teacher in her community. People spoke of her intelligence, grace, and ability. In particular, they spoke about the way her spiritual practice created a sacred feel to the classes she led. She was, in short, a yoga teacher who could create a space in which one could grow as person.

In this book, Sandy offers the reader the support she has offered the many individuals who have learned from her classes and her example over the years. She offers us guidance in three aspects of teaching.

## Character

With over twenty years of teaching experience to glean from, Sandy provides practical and relevant examples of how the developed character of a yoga teacher is one who is willing to show up well-equipped and ready to serve their community teaching yoga. Sandy understands that the heart of a yoga teacher is one that serves and connects with others while connecting others to the teachings of yoga at the same time.

## Confidence

Sandy uses the methodology of embodying the never-ending pursuit of remaining a student first in order to teach the yoga practice from a place that comes from a known experience. From confidence developed within this approach to teaching yoga, she seeks to challenge herself, and other yoga teachers, to grow beyond the initial learning phase of yoga teacher training and consistently seek to teach what must be learned. Through reflective application exercises yoga teachers can become well-equipped to step into the yoga classroom with confidence and assurance.

## Leadership

Understanding that leadership is built upon a willingness to continuously reflect and refine in order to lead from example is found within Sandy's approach and teaching methodology. This approach supports the bigger work of service to be found in sharing the practice of yoga with others and becoming an agent of change who supports their community with all that is available within the transformative lifelong practice of yoga.

It has been an honor to know Sandy and to support the work she is doing in the world. May this book bring you the peace and happiness as you work to bring Yoga into your life and the lives of those you serve.

Namaste,

*Rolf Gates*
Yoga teacher and author

# Introduction
## Why I Wrote This Book

It all begins in the heart. I stepped into my first yoga class at a crucial time in my life shortly after my mom, Iris, had passed away. I was thirty years old and a young mother of two small boys. My dad and I were my mother's primary caregivers for the last five years of her life. With her passing, my life as I had known it suddenly changed. Because of the length and severity of my mom's illness, I'd thought I was prepared for life without her, but how does anyone ever truly prepare for how abruptly life changes with the death of a loved one?

During those early, raw days of trying to figure out a new plan and a new course of action, I found myself stepping into my first encounter with the practice of yoga. I signed up for a yoga class at a local gym and quickly found that my faith and this newfound practice called yoga were going to support me through the next season of my life. Not long after I began practicing yoga, I sought out yoga teacher training. I sensed a deep desire, a stirring within, to know more about this practice, and I thought I could possibly teach a few classes while remaining a stay-at-home mom to my two preschool-aged boys.

Now, more than twenty years later, I am still teaching and sharing the practice of yoga with others. Over the years, I have continued my own quest to know more of the practice, to learn more as a student. My teaching pathway has revealed itself in a variety of ways, and I have led thousands of hours of classes, workshops, and trainings. I have also trained others to teach and thrive as yoga teachers serving their communities. Through many amazing opportunities, I have had the profound opportunity to share yoga with others who have also found themselves standing at the crossroads of life change, wondering what a yoga class might offer to them.

After teaching yoga in a variety of locations, venues, and settings, I continue to find that yoga is for everyone and that it can be shared to meet the needs of all. My vocation as a yoga teacher is to pursue a better understanding of how to meet others where they are and how to equip them with what they need on their own journey toward making peace with change. This is the heart of teaching, and this concept quickly became my motivation for teaching.

Service and connection are two facets that continue to define my approach to teaching. To share and inspire other yoga teachers to pursue this most worthy endeavor is my reason for being a yoga teacher. I have ventured into the unknown, seeking various and new ways over the years to continue to support and share yoga with others through online teaching platforms. I launched my Beyond Yoga Teacher Training Podcast in 2020, the year that brought immense change for us all.

I have come to realize there is beauty in not arriving at a conclusion, and there is still so much more to learn. Yoga teachers need an advocate and mentor in order to thrive and create longevity in teaching yoga. Along my teaching pathway, mentorship has been a vital piece of my development and growth as a yoga teacher. Teachers need mentors who can come alongside of them to advise and share from their experience in order to encourage and inspire them. I am thankful for all the mentors in my life who have supported my ongoing development as an individual and as a yoga teacher. Some have even reached out to take my hand, equipping, and guiding me to take the next step.

The quest to know more or wait until we feel like we know enough can be an obstacle for many yoga teachers. The support of a trusted mentor is necessary to evaluate and maneuver the obstacles that come along the teaching path. Because of this deep desire to support other teachers in the same capacity, I am devoted to mentoring and advocating for yoga teachers.

At the beginning of my yoga teacher training, one of my teachers and mentors, Rolf Gates, asked our training group to choose one word that would define the experience of the training for us. Gift. That was my word. The yoga practice and the opportunity to train and learn how to teach others is a gift. Not only is it a gift to myself, but it's also a gift I can continuously give to others. This gift of service filled the void I had felt within my heart when my mother passed. It was a bridge that allowed me to cross from the purposeful life I had lived caring for and serving the needs of my mother into a life of continued service sharing the practice of yoga with others.

It is my hope that this book will serve as a resource to provide guidance, encouragement, and inspiration for aspiring, new, and seasoned yoga teachers. In this book, it is important for me to share not only insight from the great lessons I have learned teaching yoga but also reflective exercises at the end of each lesson that will aid in the application and absorption of all of the teaching methodology, approaches, and techniques shared in the book. The lessons in this book are meant to provide relevance and valuable insight that supports you greatly as you step onto and move along the pathway as a yoga teacher to share and serve others with the beautiful gift of teaching yoga from your heart.

# PART ONE

# Character

# Introduction

Character is defined by the mental and moral qualities distinctive to an individual. The character of a yoga teacher extends far beyond the technical aspect of learning how to sequence a set of yoga postures. Although the techniques are important, one must also spend time exploring the deeper qualities of the mindset, motivation, and intention of practicing yoga.

## Where It All Begins

When do you know it's time to begin the journey of becoming a yoga teacher? Perhaps it begins earlier than you think. Perhaps it begins before you actually make the commitment and investment to step into your first yoga teacher training. For me, my yoga practice began with curiosity. I often say I'll try anything once — well, almost anything. On the day I found myself standing at the crossroads of a life change, I stepped into my first yoga class. I stepped in with curiosity and the notion that I needed to establish a new routine. So why not try something new?

On this particular day, I decided to do what was familiar. I went back to the gym. This day was different, though, because at the time, my morning routine consisted of working out at the gym and then taking my two toddler-aged boys with me to spend the day caring for my mom while my dad worked. My mom was diagnosed with multiple sclerosis when I was two years old, and years later, her condition had progressed to the point that she needed around-the-clock care. My dad was a small business owner, and hiring someone else to provide this level of care just was not feasible. It felt only natural that I would be the one to provide this support and care. I am grateful to my husband for his unending love and support that allowed me to step out of my role in the workforce and into the role of primary caregiver for my mom during the last five years of her life.

That day I went to the gym, though, was different. That day, I found myself seeking routine because it was my first day back to the gym after my mom had passed away. I found myself walking on the treadmill, but where was I going? Where was the monotony of walking leading me? There was now a space within me. Caring for my mom had been filling that space, and it had become a deep chasm within me. I felt empty.

As I continued to walk on the treadmill that day, I looked inside the group fitness room visible through a glass wall alongside the fitness equipment. What I saw that day intrigued me. It caught my attention, much like the yoga practice does, right? Within the depths of the chasm, I sensed a spark, a flicker of light deep within. This faint light revealed a bridge. And the light of a renewed sense of purpose called out to me, inviting me to step onto that bridge with faith and curiosity.

I felt hopeful in my ability to find yet another path of service and purpose like the one that caring for my mother had held for me. With faith, rather than the fear of the unknown, I decided to cross over. As I followed the flickering light of curiosity deep within me, I stepped onto that bridge that lead me into my first yoga class.

The heart of service that had been cultivated within me from a very young age was now beginning to see the new direction. What I came to know quickly and more fully in those early days of my yoga practice was that, all that I was and needed to move into this next phase of my life had always resided within me.

Although I had stepped onto a new, different path, I still felt a sense of familiarity. The chasm I had felt would become a space to cultivate a new way to serve others, and it would be through teaching the practice of yoga.

During those early days, when I was developing a discipline toward my personal yoga practice, it provided a great release for my grief. I found myself lying in savasana, embracing the sweet release of all the emotions within me in regard to my mom's illness. I felt relieved of the physical suffering I saw her live through, although she remained mentally calm and settled.

Despite her discomfort, pain, and ultimately the lack of being able to sense her nervous system due to the nerve and sensory damage caused by MS, my mother exuded a belief and reliance in something much bigger. I saw within her the power of positive thinking that would serve her well, and most importantly, I saw her great faith expressed in knowing that her mortal body was just that — mortal. It was perishable, but her faith and hope in the eternal would prevail. She was confident she would one day live eternally void of suffering and pain.

Perhaps this notion of service and teaching from the heart had been there all along, right in front of me. Perhaps this new season of my life and the purpose that I now sought was just a natural unfolding of what I had already lived and borne witness to through the life of my mother.

It's interesting that, as most things in life, one must experience death, or grief, of what once was in order to step into the beginning of what is to come. For me, my mother's death was the birth of the beginning of my relationship with the yoga practice and the ongoing dedication toward becoming a yoga teacher.

# The Desire to Be a Yoga Teacher

"Educating the mind without educating the heart is
no education at all."

— ARISTOTLE

As you begin your journey toward yoga teacher training, it's important to spend time in contemplation and reflection about why you even want to be a yoga teacher. Can you pinpoint what fuels this desire? It's an important question because the answer will continue to fuel you as you move along your path, and your "why" will dictate how you will go about the work and service of being a yoga teacher.

When I first started practicing yoga, a desire to teach wasn't necessarily on my radar. About six months into my journey, my teacher at that time, Susan, saw something in me that I had yet to uncover in myself. The physical aspect of yoga practice had piqued my interest in a way nothing else ever had. I had always been active, though, and exercise and physical activity had been a part of my life since I was young.

I suspect the desire to become a yoga teacher had already been percolating within me, and when that desire to connect with others in service made its way to the surface, teaching yoga felt like a natural extension of myself. In the early stages of my practice, I found a refuge and space to move through my grief after my mother's death. The practice of yoga, along with my faith practice, brought me great solace. It led me to uncover my sense of purpose once again as I faced the challenges of navigating life as a young mother without the advisement of my own mother.

In those early days, I had to sift through the emotions and thoughts of what I would now do that provided the same feeling of service as caring for my mother had. And if someone would've told me then that I would become a yoga teacher and dedicate over two decades to studying and teaching the practice, I just wouldn't have believed them. Here is where curiosity comes in again. The heart of teaching yoga comes from a heart that desires to serve and connect with others. I'll expand upon these two important elements of being a yoga teacher in the next lesson, but let's explore more deeply this simple, yet quite profound, question made up of three letters — why?

## Three Small Letters

When you explore the answer to this question, you will find where your desire to teach is rooted. If you begin to closely examine the answer and find yourself stuck on the surface of what you feel or what you think the experience of teaching yoga might be, consider whether your vision is full of self-gratification or self-service. In that case, your effectiveness as a teacher will most likely remain at the surface level, as well.

That is not to say you won't be able to dig deeper as you evolve and grow as a teacher. Within this excavation, you can discover what's available to you when you choose to teach with a confident vulnerability that allows the teachings of yoga to flow through you like a vessel pours its contents into another. It's the same when you teach from your heart.

Sometimes, as with many other areas of our lives, what

we first set out to do with the practice of yoga evolves and morphs into a different version of that original vision. This is where and why it's so important as you step out of yoga teacher training that you teach. You must teach and teach again, because it's within the real-time act of teaching that you begin to develop and learn so much about what you're teaching and what type of teacher you desire to be. Within those first couple of years of teaching, you will begin to refine and define your craft. You'll begin to develop a deeper understanding of what it means to be a yoga teacher and what this role will require of you.

As you get clear on why you're doing what you're doing, how you go about executing the technical aspect of teaching will become more clearly defined. You will revisit the question of why throughout your teaching career, because what you desire during one season in your teaching career will most likely change. You might be led to explore areas that were not what supported your quest for teaching in a past season. This is where adjusting and adapting comes in—and you do not have to fit into a specific mold as a teacher. Along the way, you'll set out to discover your unique path and gift for teaching. When you become clear on the answer of why you desire to be a yoga teacher, then your approach to teaching will mature, and teaching opportunities will manifest.

Most yoga teachers are drawn to asanas at first. As you begin to dedicate more time toward the physicality, or the doing aspect of the practice, you'll begin to notice how the various shapes and the movement in and out of the shapes create an experience. The yoga class setting becomes a space where individuals come together, each sharing in the same experience yet in a unique way.

Much can be said about the journey of being a yoga teacher.

By teaching and leading others, you will begin to notice the opportunities to create collective experiences between you, as teacher, and the students. The beauty of humanity coming together to create the experiences of life that they desire to have becomes a reality. Your role as a teacher supports this co-creation of a life where the practice of yoga lessens suffering and the essence of presence awakens within both the teacher and student. Time spent gaining clarity about your desire to teach yoga will equip you with a better understanding of how to facilitate this experience for others.

## Reflective Exercise

"Character" is defined as the mental and moral qualities distinctive to an individual. Spend a few moments evaluating the intentions, traits, and qualities already present within you that will naturally carry over into being a yoga teacher. Journal these attributes and reflect on them often, especially after leading a class. If you have just begun teaching or have not yet taught a class, then reflect upon the classes you have taken and the impact the character of the teacher had on your overall class experience.

# The Role of a Yoga Teacher: Service and Connection

"Choice is at the heart of service."
— JUDITH HANSON LASATER, YOGA TEACHER AND AUTHOR

Once you get clear on why you desire to teach yoga, it's time to define your role as a teacher. This expanded knowledge will support you further in how you will go about being a yoga teacher. The role of a yoga teacher is not as glamorous as some might envision. Still, some are drawn to the idea and the attention of being the leader where others admire and are even mesmerized by the yoga teacher. Be cautious, though, for this is the ego. Yoga teachers walk a fine line between performance and presence.

There is a slippery slope where the ego likes to creep in and confuse us within the clarity of our purpose and role as a yoga teacher. The greatest gift you can give the students you lead is being present and being real. Still, how often do we walk into yoga classes to find the teacher ready with their mat laid out as if it were a stage while they ready themselves to deliver a grand performance? Teaching yoga from the heart is an experience of humility and vulnerability rather than one fueled by ego-driven pursuits and gains.

## Service and Connection

In the pursuit of creating a sustainable teaching career with longevity, two main areas will serve as a guidepost in that pursuit: service and connection. The word yoga is derived from a Sanskrit word meaning "union" or "connection." If we're going to explore teaching from the heart, then it's important to also note and acknowledge that doing so comes from a heart acting within service to another. One of the primary roles of a yoga teacher is to serve students by unifying or connecting them with the essence and wholeness that resides in each and every one of us. Sounds simple, huh? What a grand task and responsibility as a yoga teacher! It is a most worthy endeavor to dedicate oneself to clearly understanding what is involved within this role.

To expand even further, it's through one's devoted act of service as a yoga teacher that they are able to support and impact someone else's life. The role of yoga teacher is not the role of superiority, yet it's quite the opposite. The role of yoga teacher is deeply rooted in the devotion of service that connects others to their own deep well of stillness, love and compassion. To teach yoga is to teach from a heart devoted to service. To teach yoga is to teach with and from a selfless, unattached space. To teach yoga is to teach from a heart that desires, first and foremost, to be helpful, to be of service, and to be a conduit that connects others to their own wholeness and union.

> "Therefore always perform unattached the deed to be done for the man who performs action without attachment obtains the Supreme."
> **BHAGAVAD GITA 3:19**

We are hardwired to serve, just as we are to connect with others. I'll speak more to connection in the next lesson. There are biological reasons for why we feel good when we serve others. We often think of exercise and diet as keys to living a healthier life, but research shows that social interaction, kindness, and service also contributes greatly to the quality and longevity of our lives. A pretty cool concept is that anyone can serve.

To be a yoga teacher, you need to study and develop a skill set for leading others safely and effectively through yoga asana sequences within the yoga class setting. There are definitely evaluations to be made when considering what kind of teacher you will be. Will you teach or instruct? Or will you provide a combination of both. I will discuss the difference a little later in the book. The main objective of this lesson is developing an understanding of how service and connection support and define your role and responsibilities as a yoga teacher.

## Character Traits of Service

When it comes to the act of service, it's also vital to understand what serving looks like. When serving others by teaching the practice of yoga from their heart, a yoga teacher will exhibit several important traits.

### HUMILITY

Service begins with humility. The act of giving oneself to the betterment of another requires humility. Someone who gives truly has no attachment to the gift they are giving. Humility within the act of service to another reflects and acknowledges abundance and that there is enough to go around. When it comes to yoga, there is enough to go around. There is no room for competition with another teacher or with another style of yoga. There is no room, and no time, to be given to comparison.

When you give yourself over to that competitive nature, you are taking away from that part of yourself you can give over to others in service. Competition and comparison creates a kink in the conduit that impedes your ability to provide the teachings of yoga to your students.

## SEE THE NEED

A heart of service sees needs. Yoga teacher, the greatest gift you can give the students is your presence and making them feel seen and heard within the classes you lead. To be a yoga teacher who teaches from the heart, you must recognize the needs of others and then support and help meet those needs.

In service, you support students by leading them through a yoga class experience that sets them up for success, equipping them with everything they will need to develop their own autonomy in the practice, holding nothing back. At the same time, you support students by teaching them how to practice. Facilitating the needs of a yoga class is one of your primary roles as teacher. Understanding your duty of service and the scope of care that you provide is of utmost importance so that you do not overstep when it comes to the level of service and services that you provide. Unless you have credentials and certification to provide specialized services in addition to teaching yoga, it is important that you do not increase your liability by expanding into areas of expertise that you are not equipped to provide in the yoga class setting.

## COMPASSION AND EMPATHY

Teaching from a heart of service means that you see the people beyond the poses. With compassion and empathy, you choose to see the needs of your student and address the needs of the class you're leading with the same attention you would for your own practice experience. It doesn't mean you project, or expect, others to have the same experience as you. Instead, you allow students to create the class experience they wish to have. With compassion and empathy, you connect and serve others more fully without any sense of agenda or attachment to having the practice look or be a certain way.

Teaching methodology can often become skewed when yoga teachers focus more on creating intricate and overly creative sequences while devoting too much attention to entertaining, retaining, and bringing students back to their class. By placing a priority on seeing the people first, you can more effectively evaluate how to best support the needs of those right in front of you. This attention lets students find the best shape and yoga pose that serves them that given day. This guidance might come within a set of directives and caring language that equips students with options and variations of a yoga pose that sets them up for success and safety. Meeting the needs of students with suggestions, props, or other assistance while allowing them to choose and decide what best supports their autonomy will fuel a thriving, compassionate teaching career.

## COURAGE

Serving others requires courage. You must push past your comfort zone and into unfamiliar territories in order to meet the needs of those you are serving. The role of a teacher requires courage to admit that you don't know everything and a willingness to teach what you do know while continuing to devote time to study and expanded learning. Courage also comes within a willingness to listen and seek to understand more fully what students might actually be hearing within your directives and cues. Although you may think you know what the students need, there is great courage in acknowledging that as you listen more closely you may need to adjust and adapt your approach and method for teaching.

## RESPONSIBILITY

Lastly, service requires a sense of responsibility. It's easy to get caught up with taking ownership of a class or the students who choose to practice with you. The classes you teach are not yours. You are a steward and facilitator of these experiences, but you do not own them or the students.

A sense of responsibility comes from a strong sense of community that you are part of a larger community. You also bear responsibility in cultivating and nurturing the bigger picture of the work taking place individually and collectively. If yoga is union, then by practicing yoga, you're identifying with this sense of responsibility. By teaching the practice, you acknowledge responsibility for sharing and providing instruction for others who will become a student of the practice.

## Connection

Expanding even further on the character and responsibility of service is connection. The role of a yoga teacher is to give students the opportunity to connect to the wholeness of who they are, along with others and the greater good of living a life on purpose with compassion and empathy for the elimination of suffering of all beings. When I think about connection and teaching yoga, I think about the importance of sharing the practice in a way that offers students the ability to use breath and movement in a variety of shapes to examine the interconnectedness of who they are and why they do what they do. Through the practical, yet profound, understanding of the interconnectedness and intricacies of the human body, we can begin to translate this understanding into the inner workings of our relationships with others. As yoga teachers, we can teach and lead others within this discovery through the yoga asanas and other mindfulness exercises within the yoga practice.

The yoga teacher supports this connection—it is, therefore, of great importance that a teacher understand how to do this effectively and skillfully. A skillful yoga teacher equips others with the tools and instructions to listen and move their bodies safely, while demonstrating how breath work teaches us to be present for what is and trust in what's to come. The yoga teacher equips students to notice and begin their own autonomous, intuitive excavation through the use of supportive and caring guidance, language, and clear instructions.

Once this connection is made, the yoga teacher also supports students within the discovery and cultivation of a mindset and perspective that pulls back from selfish desires in order to view the world from a larger lens. Understanding how we fit into the bigger picture of life helps us each make our own unique contribution to the overall betterment of all beings. As Brene Brown shares in one of my favorite books, *Daring Greatly*: "Connection is why we're here. We are hardwired to connect with others. It's what gives purpose and meaning to our lives, and without it there is suffering."

I find this quote most fitting for the yoga teacher. Teaching from the heart means choosing to step into the classroom to equip and connect students with the tools they will need to eliminate the habits of their minds, or the suffering. It means choosing to serve and support students, through the practice of yoga, in an ongoing pursuit or spiritual quest to find ease and elimination of suffering in their life.

## Reflective Exercise

Reflect on the Five Character Traits of Service. How does each area show up for you in your life and as a yoga teacher? Where could you place more emphasis in the classes you lead? Where could you infuse more of a trait into your interaction with students and the guidance you give as a teacher?

# Teach What You Need to Learn

---

"Never Stop Learning Because Life Never Stops
Teaching."

**— KIRILL KORSHIKOV**

Continuing to grow as a teacher is essential. This lesson discusses how the act of teaching serves as a powerful refining tool of evaluation that supports the generation of confidence teaching yoga through the concept of "teaching what you need to learn." Learn key ways you can begin to discern the areas where you need more training and deeper study within.

The concept of teaching what you need to learn represents the essence of what happens when an individual seeks to teach someone else something. This action also represents the beautiful reciprocity found within the teacher-student relationship.

It begins when you step out of YTT (yoga teacher training). First of all, you're excited—but also terrified. I know I was. You're excited to share everything you learned during training, but now you have to step out—with faith, I'll add—trust in what you do know, and teach. You'll teach to an unknown group of students who will enter the space where you'll be teaching and unroll their yoga mats with the understanding that you are going to lead them effectively through an experience that they have come seeking. This will happen whether or not students even know yet what they are seeking from the experience. Here's where the terrifying part comes in—it's no longer that comfy, warm, and fuzzy space you just spent many hours teaching in with your other like-minded trainees in your teacher training, others who were in the same position you were in. You might even feel a bit isolated and alone because you're the one in charge now. It's your time. You are solely responsible for initiating and leading the class experience.

So what do you do? It's simple — you teach. You teach from the space of what you know while also acknowledging there is much you don't know yet. And it is okay to be a new yoga teacher. It's okay to not know, because you will never really fully know it all. Hopefully, that just helped to support you with a nice long exhale.

As I mentioned earlier, students don't expect you to come in and show off and present yourself as a know-it-all or even an expert. Oftentimes, when we embark on learning something new, we have a hard time giving ourselves the space and time for learning that comes through application. I believe that students aren't looking for that at all. I know, for myself, as a student of the practice, I desire to be guided by someone who is personable, someone who "sees" the room, and someone who dedicates themselves to holding the space of the room, effectively and skillfully, with respect for all that enter the space. It's important to know your role as teacher, or leader, of the class experience.

## Hold the Space of Time

It's also important to add here, and it's something that I seek when I venture out as a student to take class, that students know they can trust you as the teacher to safeguard and protect the space of time. So please be diligent and skillful in your planning and executing of a class that begins and ends on time. This really is important. It builds trust and encourages students to release attachment to time and schedules, because they can hand that responsibility over to you.

This concept of "teach what you need to learn" can be a challenge for teachers because it requires looking more closely to the areas of our teaching skill set that may seem more subtle yet have the potential to make a really big impact within the experience we are trying to offer. Learning to hold the space of time for someone else is definitely something to work toward becoming highly efficient and skilled within. The phrase "to thine own self be true" also comes to mind here. If you know yourself and you know time management is a struggle, then I encourage you to heighten your awareness to how you structure your classes and begin to teach yourself better time management within the framework of how you sequence and lead classes.

I'll share with you a few ways that I approach this and how I've developed that internal awareness of time management that has led me to not be reliant on actually seeing the time while I'm teaching. You'll begin with the overall time that the particular class you are leading is — so I'll use an hour-long class for my example. You have sixty minutes. From there, you will need to bookend your opening and centering time of the class with the most important time of the class, which is savasana. Please, please, please do not forsake savasana or make it an afterthought in your planning. It is the key element, and you, as teacher, must safeguard this valuable portion of absorption for the students you're leading. It's important to understand that when teaching others, we tend to teach what we deem important. If you are not skillful with your time and you find yourself running out of time in a class and not giving adequate time for students to experience savasana, then you are teaching students that the ending or closing of the practice experience is not really important.

Back to my sixty-minute example. From your sixty minutes, you will then devote roughly ten percent of your class time to the opening and ten percent to savasana, at a minimum. You can certainly vary this according to your teaching emphasis that given day. The key point is to not go below that ten percent. For the sixty-minute class, you would devote six minutes to your opening and six minutes to the closing. I'll emphasize again how important savasana is and the time you spend bringing students out of savasana and closing the practice experience. Six minutes isn't going to be the progression toward savasana, rather, six minutes is going to start savasana. Now, let me also mention here that you need to be mindful of the setting and always seek to meet students where they are in regard to the final posture of savasana. You may need to break that six minutes up and instead designate a full three minutes to savasana. You can then allocate the remaining time toward a slow progression bringing students out of savasana and closing the class on time.

Realistically, learning the posture of savasana can be the most challenging for students, especially those who are new to the experience. Savasana can be unsettling and not restful, and that's okay. You still want to offer enough time for students to catch a glimpse of the experience and to build trust in their capacity to experience stillness. I say all of this because you definitely want to teach students this valuable piece of the asana practice. You also want to use discernment and meet students where they are in their learning experience without compromising because it might be a challenge for them.

I imagine you've heard students say, "I just can't be still."

You can acknowledge their observation, but don't forsake the closing of the practice experience because you want to please them.

As the teacher, you are there to lead and share with them all facets of the practice that is available and support them in finding the balance and ease within the movement and the stillness aspects of the experience.

## Teaching Anatomy

Early into my teaching, I began sensing the desire to offer more to the students I was teaching. I had become adept at leading a sequence of the postures, but I wanted to add more layers to the experience—in particular, in regard to anatomy and what I could offer students within their personal observation of what was going on in their bodies as they created the shapes that I was cueing. I knew that in order to begin learning the anatomy layer and components of the yoga asana that I would need to begin "teaching what I needed to learn."

Anatomy can be quite an overwhelming learning initiative. I quickly found that my curiosity and understanding would need to be supported by resources that were relevant for movement-based teachers, especially discussion of how the teaching of anatomy relates to yoga teachers. I began my pursuit of learning, and when it came to the application piece of the process, I approached it one pose at a time. I began to highlight one pose within the sequence of my teaching, and in that pose, I would cue and guide students within their own exploration of that particular action and anatomy emphasis I was sharing.

When it comes to learning and the ability to approach

learning without becoming overwhelmed by the vastness of a topic, simplifying the process to the learning of one pose at time really did benefit my ability to learn from what I was actually teaching. I gained invisible confidence in what I began to know from the teaching of the application through an anatomical lens. I found that this simplified approached met the needs of the students and invited them into a deeper understanding of what was taking place or what they could explore within their experience of the various yoga pose shapes. Not all students are going to be interested in hearing that guidance, but I discovered that I became a more effective teacher when I was able to go in and teach the poses along with highlighting the layers of anatomy that would then speak to a broader audience within the classes I was leading. Those who are only interested in hearing the cueing of the pose got what they were seeking, and then others were equipped with tools and focus that met their needs within the pursuits they desired from their own yoga practice. It created a wonderful layered-learning atmosphere.

## Meet Students Where They Are

During this time, I was teaching at a YMCA. When I speak to meeting the needs of the students within the various settings where we find ourselves sharing the yoga practice, it's important to note that the approach could be less about presenting a deep dive into the philosophical teachings of yoga, especially in an environment focused more on physical fitness, such as a YMCA or a gym. You have the choice. As a teacher, you can decide what you will share. As part of my journey as a teacher, I desire to share as much of the experience of the practice of yoga as I can while still meeting people where they are.

This includes considering how much they want to devote to a deeper understanding of the practice of yoga.

I have also taught in yoga studios, and I think it's important to place yourself in a variety of settings to teach. This afforded me great opportunities to expand and grow as a teacher. I will say that I approached my classes at the Y with a mindset to lead an experience that didn't hold back from my students. I didn't solely lead an experience from the physical aspect just because it was in a fitness setting. I wanted to provide the students at the YMCA an experience just like I would in the yoga studio setting. It was also very important to me that I remain an approachable and accessible teacher, to support all students so that they could discover what they were seeking and in their own timing, regardless of where they were practicing.

I knew that some students at the YMCA would most likely never walk through the doors of a yoga studio, and that did not matter. I wanted to offer students all facets and layers of the experience so that it would add to their journey through the various yoga classes at the YMCA, regardless of whether I was the teacher. I knew there were anatomy and subtle energetic aspects of what takes place within the asana practice that are beyond the physicality of the practice. My focus was to provide students with the tools and teaching emphasis that might pique their curiosity down the road.

## Restraint and Trust

Lastly, when it comes to teaching what you need to learn, I want to emphasize that in order to be an effective and skillful teacher, you do not have to be all things to all students. It is okay to stay in your lane. It is easy to become swept up and distracted, bouncing from one training to the next while consuming as many trainings as you can with the hopes that when you accumulate a collection of trainings, you will become the teacher you desire to be. I highly encourage you to teach first. Teach what you know and then spend time listening and observing your own experiences as a teacher. You will learn so much of what it means to be a teacher through the act of simply teaching.

You don't need to run around town or across the globe, seeking the next latest-and-greatest training. It takes a huge amount of restraint to be with yourself where you currently are in your teaching, developing trust in what you do know that comes through the application of teaching. Put yourself out there and teach in a variety of settings that will challenge you to relate and grow as a teacher. What I have come to know after over two decades of teaching experience is that what you need to learn will arise within the act of teaching. Listen closely to those little moments of curiosity and then seek to refine and learn from the simplicity of a lens that isn't overwhelmed with trying to replicate or become something you aren't or by trying to overload yourself with knowledge without applying all that you do know first.

Listen to the promptings of your own intuitive intelligence. It will not let you down or steer you toward something inauthentic—your ego will do that, so be cautious and discern between the two. When you look outside yourself and think that becoming a successful teacher requires you to replicate or pursue what other teachers are doing, that is a red flag. Your ego has crept in within the masquerade of imposter syndrome, and that indicates it is time to refocus and realign yourself with the bigger aspect of why you became a yoga teacher in the beginning. I'll speak more to imposter syndrome in lesson nine, as well as the competition and collaboration with other teachers in lesson ten.

Once you realign with your purpose—which you will do repeatedly within your vocation as a yoga teacher I might add—then how you pursue your distinct teaching path will clearly reveal itself. Within that discernment, you will begin to know whether another training is necessary. You will then dive into that authentic pursuit and begin absorbing and applying what you're learning, and the process and cycle of teaching what you need to learn will repeat itself.

Being a yoga teacher is truly a worthy endeavor. Is it easy? No. It is certainly worth the effort, though. My desire is that you know who you are as a teacher and that you challenge yourself to grow and refine as you seek to share the beautiful gift of yoga with as many individuals as possible. No one can teach like you because no one else is uniquely you. Go out and share your gift and teach what you need to learn along the way.

## Reflective Exercise

Evaluate which areas of your teaching skill set that you would like to develop and learn more about. Seek to expand your knowledge in these areas while beginning to actually teach the concepts of subject matter you desire to understand better.

# Identity Crisis of a New Yoga Teacher

---

"The spiritual energy released by our practice strips
away all that is false, the way a wind blows sand from
the surface of a mirror."

**– ROLF GATES, YOGA TEACHER AND AUTHOR**

The love of practicing yoga most likely drew you to become a yoga teacher, but beware of imbalance when you begin to teach more than you practice. In this lesson, understand how your personal practice time is integral and naturally infused into your development as a teacher and the importance of remaining consistent with your personal practice time.

An identity crisis happens at a time when change makes you re-evaluate who you are. Most likely, we can all relate or have experienced an identity crisis at some point in our lives. What about the moment you step out of yoga teacher training? Perhaps you're reading this and you have just begun teacher training or have been contemplating pursuing a teacher training. Imagine with me for a moment how it is going to feel when you complete the training and you graduate and receive your certificate of completion from yoga teacher training.

Envision the completion of your training experience. Perhaps, you have already actually experienced the completion of your YTT experience. Either way, in that moment, you will most likely experience various swirling of emotions, possibly even doubt and wonder. And the thought of what comes next is often in your thoughts. You may have felt frozen, fearful even, of the unknown and unsure what direction you should take to do this thing called teaching yoga. What had just began to feel comfortable within your training experience has now shifted to the realization that it's now showtime and all that you have studied and hopefully began to absorb has now shifted into the foreground.

The moment you complete teacher training, there is a realization that the rubber is hitting the road and it is go time. Within the various yoga teacher trainings that I have lead, I always strongly encourage trainees to continue teaching immediately once the training is over. Don't take a break. Keep teaching. The teaching practicum aspect of a two-hundred-hour foundational teacher training is crucial. I have always focused heavily on getting trainees set up and teaching from the very beginning of the training and within the very first weekend of YTT. After all, it is a teacher training, right?

Now, getting back to new teachers—and it's possible you completed YTT a while ago but never really dove into teaching after the training experience and may feel a bit unsettled, or even new when it comes to teaching. Rather than feeling like you must roll out of YTT and take on a new identity, I want to encourage you to meet yourself where you are and give yourself some space and grace to be new at something. And in particular, give yourself permission to be a new yoga teacher. Being new at something is a beautiful learning space, so don't miss it or try to bypass it, trying to hurry yourself along within the process of developing and growing as a teacher. Interestingly, this season of being new is part of the growing process, and if you desire to create sustainability and longevity in this vocation of service as a yoga teacher, then I'm going to highly encourage you to get comfortable in this developmental area. You will quickly find, if you haven't already, that there is so much to learn and there is beauty in the process of realizing there is no arrival at knowing all there is to know about the practice of yoga and teaching.

## The Process of Learning

I want to begin by addressing the concept of learning and shine some light on what happens when we venture into a new learning experience. From my experience, new teachers might feel a spectrum of emotions from excitement to terror, all at the same time when deciding to learn something new. Here's where trusting the process and being in the process comes in again.

I can remember the very first class I taught. I had been practicing yoga for a while. I had spent time in a training, and I had prepared my sequence for the class. Still, I felt a flood of extreme fear right before the class began. I could've easily turned around and decided that teaching was not for me, but I did it anyway. And I'm so glad I did. It was my starting point, and as I share this experience with you today, well over twenty years later, I can still see the room and remember the scene vividly.

Learning a new skill is often an extremely rewarding experience. Venturing into a YTT to learn how to share and teach yoga provides you with a wonderful opportunity to first dive into your own personal understanding and experience of the yoga practice. And then there is the quest to learn how to express, communicate, share, and teach others by equipping them with the tools they will need to venture into their own discovery within the yoga practice. How fulfilling is that? At the same time, though, an ongoing pursuit of learning must take place, and as I've already mentioned, there is no arriving because there will always be fresh and new ways to learn and encounter the practice of yoga based upon your developed understanding and application of the practice.

Why do we rush the process, though? We get caught up in expectations and attachments to how we had envisioned this role of being a yoga teacher would be. We get swept up in the identity — or the "identity crisis," I'll call it. We even find ourselves disappointment because teaching yoga requires a lot more effort than we realized when we signed up for YTT. Somehow, we misunderstood what would be asked of us. Somehow, it seemed like it should be easier than this because of the great love of yoga you have.

If it were that easy, though, would it really have the rewarding impact that learning this new skill of teaching yoga has to offer? Even after twenty years, I remain committed to learning and expanding my knowledge and experience of the practice so that I can share with others more effectively and skillfully. To learn is to explore, to go beyond what you thought you understood and to commit and dedicate yourself to embarking upon the discovery consistently.

## Be Where You Are

If you are new to teaching yoga, I want to encourage you to be just that — a new teacher. There is great beauty in being where you are rather than attempting to fake it until you make it or trying to replicate what other teachers are doing. The concept of being who you are and recognize being where you are in your developmental season as a teacher applies to all teachers, regardless of how long you've been teaching.

Part of your development as a new teacher comes within the practical and real time experiences of actually teaching.

In this stage, you take all that you were equipped with and what you learned in YTT, and you begin to apply it through the act of teaching. You may have heard the phrase, "When one teaches, two learn." There is great truth in this statement.

In the beginning, your classes might feel clunky as you begin to apply all that you learned and are continuing to learn by actually leading others through a yoga class. Remind yourself it's okay to be new. Students are not expecting perfection, and it's unrealistic to place that heavy load on yourself. You will learn to refine your teaching methodology and approach, whether it's how you are sequencing or what you are offering as guidance with your language and cue directives. When your teaching feels clunky, notice and make adjustments for the next class. I call these "next time" mental notes.

## Simplify the Process

A dear friend and teacher mentee, Dominique, shared with me about a teaching experience she had where she felt and experienced this clunkiness I'm talking about. She felt that there was just something off within the class experience she had lead. After some reflection, she realized her approach to sequencing in that class was too complex. From this observation, Dominique chose to lead the next class she taught through a progression of the same sequence, offering simplicity and repetition with the culmination of a final sequence that had been built upon this layered approach and progression of sequencing. Ultimately, this approach lead to a wonderful collective experience that allowed her to call the poses then step back and bear witness to a beautiful masterpiece being created right in front of her. She felt more connected, and, more importantly, she sensed the students felt connected in the overall experience, as well. This is a wonderful example of using those less-than-seamless teaching moments as opportunities to evaluate and refine the next teaching experience.

The clunky teaching moments aren't only for those who are new to teaching, either. I still occasionally encounter those moments and make those mental "next time" markers to adjust for the next class.

## Give Yourself Some Grace

What does it mean to give yourself grace? Giving yourself grace is giving yourself permission to move along and grow from what you might consider a mistake or a less-than-enjoyable teaching experience. Will you go into every class you lead and deliver a seamless and well-articulated class? No. So why do we put that much pressure on ourselves? Well, here's where that identity crisis comes in.

We are trying to be perfect. We are trying to be something that is just not attainable. Now, I do want to add here that this is not an excuse to become the teacher who is known for always dropping a pose or the one who never knows where they are in a sequence. It is important that you seek to develop and grow in your efficiency of delivering a class experience that maintains and connects others within a steady stream and flow of one-pointed awareness. It is important to evaluate where your obstacles are when it comes to particular areas of your teaching skill set and pursue a growth strategy that supports your development in these areas.

When it comes to teaching, when you release the attachment of perfection and focus more on your presence as a facilitator in the classroom, then it takes the pressure off you and gives students a greater opportunity to learn and develop a deeper understanding of the practice of yoga for themselves.

Here's where part of the culprit of the identity crisis comes in when you buy into the concept that you must deliver a well-crafted and creative yoga pose sequence every time in order to be worthy of being a yoga teacher. I think that quite possibly what trips us up is that we have been inspired by other teachers along our yoga practice journey, and we may even venture into teacher training with some notion that we'll come out of it replicating or teaching just like the great teachers who have encouraged and inspired our passion and desire to teach. We overlook the fact that this process is not about becoming something or someone else. Rather it is always about you being you and discovering the great teacher already within you.

So, how do you uncover this? Well, you begin at the beginning. Start with your personal practice. This is so important in your development as a teacher. You practice to gift yourself the practice rather than practicing solely in preparation to teach—there is a difference. If you desire to grow and expand as a teacher, you will need to remain dedicated to your personal practice time. You will need to go beyond and below the surface and venture from the exterior aspects of what we visualize the yoga practice to be and move into the interior to experience a fresh encounter of the practice for ourselves. You will then be able to discern how to show up and hold the space for others, as a teacher, so that they might have their own fresh encounter.

Teachers often approach me about feeling discontented with teaching or feeling uninspired and lacking in this fresh encounter I've just mentioned. The first question I ask is "How is your personal practice time?" Many respond that it has diminished. Many are teaching a lot and have found it hard to carve out time for their personal practice. For some, personal practice time is non-existent, which is a huge red flag to notice. I believe that for many yoga teachers, there is even a misconception that your personal practice time is the time you spend toward preparing to teach. This can be subtle, tricky, and misleading. In order to stay aligned within your purpose and authentic identity as a teacher, you will need to remain dedicated to your personal practice time. This is your time. This is not time that you are devoting to the act of teaching, although this time will, no doubt, spill over into your teaching. Your personal practice will inspire your teaching.

## The Story Leaves out the Process

As I wrap up this lesson, I want to acknowledge that each of us has a story of how we came to first know and encounter the yoga practice. As yoga teachers, we also have a story of what inspired us to step into teacher training. Too often, though, we forget the process of learning that took place, and is required, for us to actually apply what we are learning. We forget the valuable application and absorption time that is crucial to the process. We try to jump over the process and arrive at some end point of completion or mastery before we've even put the effort or hours into developing our craft and our unique understanding and approach to teaching.

I want to encourage you to trust the process and to stay in the process. Be wary of the ego when it arises to convince you otherwise. Being new at anything is a great place to be. Being a new yoga teacher is a beautiful acknowledgment of being willing and vulnerable to show up and do the work to continue to grow and refine in your skill set of teaching. There is no need to try to replicate someone else's skills. Lastly, keep learning, keep believing, and keep being willing to discover and grow into the beautiful teacher already within you.

## Reflective Exercise

Designate a specific time daily for your personal practice time. Commit to this time and then journal your experience. Notice when your teaching mind took over or distracted you from the experience of learning and being a student.

# Style or Substance

---

"I cannot teach anybody anything; I can only make them think."

**– SOCRATES**

You have a choice as to what type of teacher you will be. In this lesson, discover the implications of choosing style over substance and what steps you will take to define the choice in your development. In this lesson, we'll explore how your approach to teaching impacts what you will share about the practice of yoga in the classes that you lead.

The methods you use to teach classes are the how of the process of learning, but oftentimes, we can get so caught up in the how, or the style, that we fail to grasp the why behind our choice of actions. As you venture out into the world of teaching after your YTT, a solid foundation based on knowing why you teach will benefit you greatly. It will influence the substance, the framework of cueing, and sequencing the classes you lead.

Teaching effectively is more than just grouping a series of yoga pose shapes together. Nothing is random when it comes to sequencing. There is an intuitive intelligence that is to be infused within the art of sequencing. In order to create, or co-create, a masterpiece of a yoga class experience, then your approach to sequencing and your understanding of this aspect is vital.

Let's explore now the concept of your overall teaching

methodology in regard to getting clearer on what type of teacher you will choose to be. Methodology matters greatly because it impacts your overall approach to teaching and determines whether you will be a teacher of substance or perhaps a teacher of style.

Methodology is defined as "a system of methods used in a particular area of study or activity." Can you clearly state what your methodology is when it comes to leading a yoga class? If you can't now, no worries. By the end of the lesson, you will be more equipped in your evaluation and begin to align into the clarity of the decision you'll make in this area.

Clarity and understanding are important when it comes to knowing why you even desire to teach yoga and to be a yoga teacher. I believe that when it comes to yoga teacher training, there is a big myth, or misconception, that you will magically turn into an experienced teacher at the end of the training period. It sounds too far-fetched to actually believe, right? Yet, this "Cinderella experience" traps many new teachers.

Besides a love of yoga, being a yoga teacher requires work—a lot of work actually. It's important that you're passionate about what you're going teach. However, it's equally important that you commit to doing the work necessary to make teaching a successful experience for you… and for the students you lead in class.

## Practicing Yoga Versus Teaching Yoga

Practicing yoga and teaching yoga are two totally different experiences. I want to touch on a couple of areas that will hopefully support you within this quest for clarity. Once you begin to get clear in your understanding, it will be easier to add a layer of ease to the effort you'll commit to teaching yoga.

Two approaches take place in the yoga class setting. Although I'll speak distinctly to the two approaches as if they are separate, I also want to emphasize that we can experience both approaches together in the collective experience of a yoga class. It's important to evaluate your approach, because it will impact how you show up in your role in the yoga classroom.

## TEACHER-CENTERED APPROACH

Within the teacher-centered methodology, the teacher provides active instruction or presentation, and the student passively receives that information from the instructor. Basically, the teacher imparts a set of directives and instructions, and students implement what they are being directed to do. I'll dig into the difference between being a yoga instructor and being a yoga teacher in the next lesson. As teachers, we all have a distinct teaching methodology, and it's important that you take time to define and understand yours better so that you lessen any confusion about your role in the yoga classroom.

## STUDENT-CENTERED APPROACH

Within the student-centered methodology, the process of learning is a collaborative effort—or co-creation, as I like to call it. Students learn and ultimately create their unique, autonomous experience within the class setting. The teacher models and acts as a facilitator, I liken the role to being a facilitator of flow, providing and facilitating an experience with directives that invite curious exploration and empowered choices. The student ultimately chooses how they want to learn in the experience and how they will go about learning from their unique practice experience while still remaining under the guidance and supervision of the teacher.

The main difference between teacher-centered and student-centered approach is that within teacher-centered approach, students focus completely on the teacher, whereas in a student-centered classroom, both students and teachers have equal focus, and the mission is a collaborative, co-created experience. When the approach is more teacher-centered, students passively explore what the teacher has imparted and offered. The experience remains solely within the realm of the experience that the teacher came in to provide. I'll note here, too, that this approach heightens the chance of a projected experience being placed on the students and the students' focus diminishing as they possibly begin to subconsciously follow the teacher rather than make choices based upon their own assessments and needs.

## What's the difference?

I'm highlighting both approaches so that you can become better informed on how you approach teaching or leading a yoga class. I'll be careful not to reflect one approach as good or better—but there is a difference. It's important that you understand the difference because it will impact your methodology, your teaching experience, and the type of teacher you will become.

Let's consider three particular areas of evaluation and focus when it comes to defining your teaching methodology. Within these three areas, I'll discuss them as opposites. It is my hope that within evaluating the difference between the two that you'll begin to also notice how this shows up in your approach to teaching. I often find that in order to know what something is more fully that an important learning component is to know what it's not.

## RELEVANCE VERSUS INCONSEQUENTIAL

First, I've found that when something in my life provides relevance, there is a greater opportunity and likelihood of a lastly effort being made toward my continuation of that activity or pursuit. On the other hand, when something seems insignificant or inconsequential, it is less likely to remain part of my daily routine.

I think this is an important designation to consider in your approach and overall teaching methodology. It speaks greatly to how you organize and sequence your classes. Are the class plans and sequences that you are offering providing relevance for your students? Is your approach to sequencing focused more on creativity and unusual movement patterns and progressions, or do you organize your classes within a structured plan that moves students sequentially and intelligently though their bodies, where they can find relevance for daily living through the practice experience that the asana sequences are providing them? It's important to note the functional piece of sequencing when it comes to relevance of our overall class plans. Are you providing students with an opportunity to develop functional awareness within the yoga asana shapes on the yoga mat and supporting them in translating its relevance to their daily lives?

Students find relevance in living their yoga outside the yoga class setting. They remember and apply the experience they create in the yoga class out in their world, and through this created experience, they find relevance for daily living through the discipline of their yoga practice. Does your current teaching methodology have substance? Does the why that backs your teaching reflect relevance within the classes you lead?

## DESCRIPTIVE VERSUS PRESCRIPTIVE

A descriptive approach implies analysis and adaptation, whereas a prescriptive approach implies what one should do. What are your initial thoughts about these two words as they are applied within the context of teaching a yoga class?

I think the biggest observation I notice within the classes that I've taken is that many teachers are approaching teaching through a prescriptive lens. You can even hear it with the choice of words they use to direct and lead the class experience. This might sound like, "I want you to _____" or "You should feel this _____." Sounds subtle, right? But the implications behind these statements express much more, and these small words make a significant impact on how you approach teaching.

Once again I want to be very clear here: you can certainly teach from this approach. My intent is not to be prescriptive in telling you what I think you should or should not do or how you should or shouldn't teach. Rather, my intent is to pique your curiosity to observe and evaluate your approach and get clear on the impact that various approaches will make on the learning environment.

As you step out onto the pathway to teach and as you begin to accumulate teaching experience, there is a time when it will benefit you greatly to take full responsibility for the type of teacher you will be and to seek ongoing clarity for what you teach and why you teach it. The mark of maturation for a yoga teacher is choosing for yourself what your approach will be. The responsibility is yours to decide and to be in an ongoing quest of development, absorbing and applying all that you glean from your teaching experiences. In this regard, your teaching experiences will truly become yours. They will be a reflection of you rather than a replication of an experience or imitating how you think you should be as a teacher.

## INDEPENDENCE VERSUS DEPENDENCE

This can be a tricky one. If you aren't careful, you could possibly be teaching students dependence and attachment to you. Once again, this approach falls mostly into that teacher-centered approach. What's happening in this situation is that the teacher is active instructing the class and presenting the sequence they have prepared with possibly minimal space for adaption or adjustments.

This type of approach could also present itself as the teacher staying solely on their yoga mat, practicing as they teach (I use the word "teach" loosely here). This can be your approach to teaching. It is more instructing at this point, and you will likely miss a great opportunity to educate and deepen the learning experience by stepping off your mat and responding to what's actually taking place in the room.

In this set of contrasting words of evaluation, independence applies not only to the approach of teaching students but also to you as the teacher. You can certainly remain dependent upon a set sequence with the same rote cues while staying firmly planted on your mat. This can create a learning experience where students are dependent upon their need to "see" you to know where they "should" be going in the practice — this takes them outside of noticing their experience. It makes them reliant, even attached, to you and your experience of the practice.

Alternatively, you can choose independence by stepping off your mat and trusting yourself as you step out into the freedom of teaching the real-time encounter that's right in front of you. If I sound like I'm highly encouraging you to pursue this approach of independence, it's because I'm doing exactly that. From my experience, the moment I chose this approach many years ago, it expanded my awareness and methodology like nothing else. It has made a lasting change in me as a teacher and in my approach to teaching. It's a change for the better, and I wouldn't want to approach teaching in any other way.

The concept and experience of teaching from this approach and methodology provides a beautiful opportunity to experience the working of something much bigger. This approach has given way to teaching experiences that truly align within service and connection to others. This approach is expansive and less restrictive than an approach where we remain in the recall space of our minds, giving prescriptive instructions. Most importantly, it fulfills the call to service and connection within the co-creative experience in the setting of a yoga class. For these reasons, I want all teachers to better understand why they teach and that the how, the choice of style or substance, within teaching methodology does matter.

## Analysis and Adaptation

Lastly, let's talk about analysis and adaptation. These two words explore the student-centered approach more deeply. When you teach off your mat and are immersed in the room, you will analyze what you see and, from that assessment, begin to offer directives and cues that address the real-time needs or adaptations of class participants. Now, it is necessary, especially when you begin teaching, to have planned sequences and a catalog of go-to cues.

Here's where responsibility comes in—there will come a

time in your teaching experiences when you'll find yourself at a crossroads. Will you choose to dig deeper, to explore and understand a more substantial aspect of teaching yoga or will you remain on the surface of the style of the experience?

You can decide to stay where you are, teaching the same sequence and the same set of cues and hope that the directives that you've memorized will serve and meet the needs of the students. And they will—to some extent. At the crossroads, though, you will be presented with a choice of faith, really. Do you have faith in and trust yourself to analyze, discern, and make adaptations to your approach to teaching that include the pulling away from certainty in what you learned in YTT and step into what feels like unfamiliar territory. It will be uncomfortable at first, but this where you begin to teach what you need to learn. As you develop within this uncomfortable, unknown space, you will become disciplined as a teacher finding the confidence and assurance that will keep you moving forward in what will become an expanded version of yourself as a yoga teacher. It's your choice.

If you are already a yoga teacher, I encourage you to keep teaching. Keep evaluating and seeking the expansion of your understanding of the practice. Keep practicing and remain faithful to being a student of the practice. Your best preparation to teach will come not solely from the time you devote to preparing class sequences but will also come from your personal practice time. If you're contemplating a yoga teacher training, then keep exploring and seek out the best fit for you. Not all trainings are created equally, and it will serve you well to spend time evaluating various programs to better understand their focus when it comes to teaching methodology.

## Reflective Exercise

Take a moment to journal what you envision a yoga teacher to look like, along with the attributes of character of someone who teaches yoga. Reflect upon this perceived image. How does this image impact your desire to teach? How does this image impact others?

# Yoga Teacher or Yoga Instructor

---

"The mediocre teacher tells. The good teacher
explains. The superior teacher demonstrates. The
great teacher inspires."

– WILLIAM ARTHUR WARD

Are you a yoga teacher… or are you a yoga instructor? There is a difference. This lesson will uncover the differences between being a yoga teacher who teaches and one who instructs. In this lesson, explore the similarities between both approaches. You most likely will blend the two approaches to build your overall approach.

## Teacher or Instructor

Let's begin by defining the terms "teacher" and "instructor." I like to google and explore definitions from various sources to get a clearer understanding of the meaning of the words that I use. I think often we interchange words when there is far more depth that can redefine how we interpret and use words once we know the distinct implications behind each word. Such is the case with the words "teacher" and "instructor." The word instructor is defined as "someone who teaches something, usually a technical skill."

A teacher is defined as "someone who helps people to learn." A teacher facilitates and supports an environment for learning, as well. Google search results for the word teacher describe some qualities of a "good teacher." These include skills in communication, listening, collaboration, adaptability, empathy and patience. Other characteristics of effective teaching included an engaging classroom presence, value in real-world learning, exchange of best practices, and a love of lifelong learning. I'll also add that a great teacher inspires others to cultivate and access these qualities within the environment of the experience they are facilitating.

Take a moment and pause to evaluate your personal experiences with individuals who have instructed you or taught you in the yoga practice. Was there a difference between these experiences? Until now, you may have felt that the words "instructor" and "teacher" were interchangeable.

I believe we see this represented in this interchangeable way within the yoga studios or spaces where we practice. I also believe these terms can get muddied. The difference is worth exploring so that you can begin to better understand the role, responsibility, and identity you will align with as a yoga teacher... or a yoga instructor.

When I explored these two terms, I found overlap, as well as subtle, yet profound, differences. One noticeable point of difference is that instructors teach a specific practical skill, whereas teachers impart theoretical knowledge of a subject or area of study rather than its practical application. Interestingly, I also want to note that I ran across an illustration that suggested that there are distinctions between the two terms and, importantly, the specific distinction that a teacher can perform the role of an instructor although an instructor cannot perform the role of a teacher. Have you ever consider this?

Deeper yet, you can teach someone something then give them instructions so that they know about it or know how to perform the specific activity or objective. This adds even more to the concept that the teacher can perform the role of instructing others on what I like to call "the how." You might even consider that a teacher is someone who teaches someone something that inspires them to explore their thoughts, feelings, and/or actions in a new or different way. Teachers offer guidance and instruction into a new perspective within the learning experience. When we teach a yoga class, we are not only providing an experience but also equipping and teaching others how to practice yoga.

I almost prefer the word facilitator to better describe my role as a yoga teacher. In the yoga practice experience, I am facilitating an environment for others to learn from their own unique, autonomous experience. Perhaps I am even instructing them in how to do this. I often consider whether we can ever really teach anyone anything. Instead, aren't we facilitating a learning environment where others can come to know or teach themselves?

## Establishing an Identity

It's important to spend time strengthening your understanding of your established identity as a yoga teacher. If we aren't evaluating this aspect of our role, then we could begin to view ourselves solely as instructors leading yet another movement-based modality. We instruct students on how to perform the yoga asana shapes with heightened emphasis placed most often upon the physicality aspect rather than the intertwined acknowledgment of the environment of learning that comes beyond the physical layers of the practice experience.

This is often expressed by the "teacher" leading the class from their own mat by demonstrating and instructing the physical layer more heavily than the relational aspect. Teachers instead seek to offer guidance in the creation of a fuller experience accessed within the more subtle layers of exploration that deepens the learning students' experience.

At this point, consider whether remaining on the mat, even practicing along with the students, is really teaching. You are certainly demonstrating and giving instructions, but this might not be teaching. If you remain on your mat, you are most likely not seeing the needs of the students right in front of you. Moving about the practice space allows you to see the students and meet them in the present moment, attending to their needs. Remember, the instructor does not teach, while the teacher's role is to teach and instruct.

## Get Off of Your Mat and Into the Room

I highly encourage you to develop the skill of teaching from off your mat. There is certainly a time and place for offering demonstrations, but the class experience does not require you to be on your mat, demonstrating, the entire time. I am a huge advocate for this approach to teaching for many reasons. Primarily, it is so that you might see and meet the needs of the room and the students, and that you might elevate the experience you are facilitating. Remaining on your mat creates a disconnect that separates you from the students. When you are not immersed in the practice space, your ability to offer guidance and support diminishes, and you begin to teach from a rote space rather than a real-time space of reading the energy of the room and providing instruction from the present moment.

Let me ask you this—do you translate teaching a yoga class into an opportunity for you to practice? And would this approach align with the aspect of service when it comes to teaching yoga? I understand that there is great vulnerability in stepping off the mat and into the room, to teach. It requires great trust in yourself that you do have the knowledge and you have all you need to lead the next posture in the sequence. I promise you that the moment you commit to getting off your mat to teach, that you will change as a teacher. You will shift from instructing to teaching. The experience of teaching off the mat will give you freedom. It will free you from the constructs of your mind, which would otherwise remain in the left-brain recall-and-recite space, and shift you more into the development of the relational right-brained aspect. And when you combine the technical left-brain function with the relational right-brain function, then essentially, you begin to teach and share from a full-brained experience within your mind. That's pretty amazing, isn't it?

You will find yourself open to a newly organized space that allows you to teach from seeing, assessing, and guiding from what is actually taking place in real time rather than what you might think is happening when you instruct solely from the confined space of your yoga mat.

I want to encourage you to explore this approach right away. If you are newer to teaching, then the transition might not seem so abrupt or scary. If you've taught for a while and remained solely on your mat while doing so, then I understand that this concept and new approach could seem daunting and unattainable. I want to assure you that you are capable. Start small. Choose small increments of time in the class when you will explore stepping off your mat. For example, teach the sequence on one side and then leave your mat to teach the second side within the practice space, cueing and leading from what you are seeing. With repetition and commitment to this new approach, you will begin to notice and feel the difference in teaching approaches. You will begin to embrace the connection and attentive energy that teaching off your mat will offer not only to your students but to you, as well.

I do to not want to dismiss the expertise of instructors, the knowledge of asana, or their benefits. A teacher may rarely spend time instructing from their mat unless a demonstration is needed and will enhance the learning experience. Demonstrations can be given from any area of the room. A teacher uses great discernment in understanding when this contribution should be made so that it doesn't become a distraction that draws students away from the interior of the practice experience. Demonstrations should be thoughtfully used as an added layer of visual learning but not last long enough to diminish students' focus. If not careful, students will begin to subconsciously follow the teacher's demonstration, diminishing the development of their own autonomous practice.

## Facilitators of Flow

When it comes to offering visual demonstrations, if you have a room full of beginners, then it will naturally be necessary for you to provide a visual demonstration and allow the initial learning aspect of the practice to begin. Once you've been able to establish consistency with a beginners group, then you will want to begin equipping them to practice using their own abilities and capacity for remembering as you heighten their learning process by stepping off the mat. You can then rely on the clarity of your cues and language to communicate the movements and allow them the process of deepening their learning experience.

Going back to the meaning of the word "facilitator" — as yoga teachers, we should be mindful that a huge aspect of teaching yoga is supporting students in establishing a rhythmic flow that resides in the present moment of awareness and supporting them in sustaining a one-pointed concentrated effort of awareness. As facilitators of this flow, we want to be mindful that our teaching methods and approaches do not hinder or "break the flow." And when the instruction or demonstration pulls students away from that flow state of awareness, then teachers should seek to quickly refocus the experience back to the flow state. Clear visual and audible guidance will support this. If one-pointed focus and the awareness and remembrance of being present is of importance to yoga teachers, then teachers will need to remain aware and conscious, themselves, of the continual emphasis to not diminish this effort.

Much of teaching yoga is about meeting the needs of students using your skill set, technically and relationally, to offer a highly effective and successful experience. This success can be measured by the students' ability to remember on their own. As a teacher, you are going to commit to reminding students until they indeed remember.

Should you need to demonstrate or "workshop" a particular posture or transition, then it's also your responsibility to quickly return to facilitating the experience after demonstrating. Within this responsibility, you see again where and how the directives you're offering are being received and applied. Another important aspect of becoming an effective yoga teacher is developing a cueing vocabulary and language that is so clear and direct that you will begin to say less and students can begin to accomplish more.

Just as your visual demonstrations should not be a distraction, it's of great importance that your cues and language are clear and direct. Ultimately, the initiation of the action you are inviting is what you seek. If you aren't seeing that, then it's your responsibility, not the student's, to adjust and adapt to find the right cue and language that produces the desired response. A key aspect of effective communication is to consider and evaluate what students might actually be hearing or interpreting from the cues and language you use to lead the class. This is where the importance again comes of being off your mat and in the room so that you can see better how your cues and language are being received — or not received.

## Attention and Intention

Where do you place your attention when it comes to preparing to lead a yoga class? What is your intention for the students you lead? These two questions are great inquiries to make as you evaluate the type of teacher you desire to be and what you will teach students.

Begin with your own personal practice. Observe and evaluate your relationship with the yoga practice. Ultimately, as a yoga instructor or teacher, you will teach or share from your own personal experience of yoga and the interpretation of the practice. This adds another piece of observation to the role of yoga teacher. In your personal learning and ongoing study, be sure that you are spending time evaluating your perspective and seeking different lenses, as well, to view the practice. Stay dedicated to your personal practice time and venture out to take different class styles and practice under the guidance of other teachers. Most importantly, remain a student always.

Be authentic to your own understanding, and this will support you greatly in your role as a yoga teacher. If you consider yourself more of an instructor, then devote yourself to the technical aspect of understanding the how of the practice. If you consider yourself more of a teacher, then devote time to understanding how to better facilitate and instruct the doing aspect while incorporating the space for the teachings of yoga to be shared, exploring the more subtle being aspect that layers beyond the how of instruction of the physical aspect of the yoga practice.

What will be your approach when you lead a class? Part of your role and responsibility as a teacher is to create a safe learning environment for students while also seeing and meeting the needs that arise during that experience. There are layers of responsibilities built into your role as a teacher that go beyond the technical ability to skillfully create sequences. That aspect is important. However, the bigger aspect of creating a learning environment where students feel seen and equipped to grow allows for the cultivation of a sustainable and consistent practice that supports the relevance of daily living.

## Developing Trust Between the Student-Teacher Relationship

Your attention to providing a safe, inclusive, and accessible learning environment and seeing and meeting the needs of the students will increase trust. This allows students a better opportunity to also develop one-pointed awareness and sustain concentrated effort.

A yoga class is an experiential learning environment rather than a setting where students are observing the practice or expertise of the teacher and their skill set. Teaching is not a performance, and the greatest gift we can offer students is our attentive presence in holding this safe, and sacred, space for them. This is where service and connection meet once again in the bigger picture of your role as a yoga teacher.

## Quality of Experience

Whether instructor or teacher, when you define your role and understand your responsibilities more clearly, you will become more effective and skillful within your role. When you are clear, you invite students into the same understanding of clarity in their role. Ultimately, your clarity will elevate the experience not only for students but also for yourself and your continued growth and desire for ongoing effectiveness leading and sharing the yoga practice.

Lastly, what you call yourself isn't really in question here. Your ability to refine and grow as a yoga teacher is dependent upon your understanding of your identity and the impact of your role. You can totally seek to develop your technical skill set for instructing others within the physicality of the yoga asana and their function. If you desire to deepen the teaching aspect of your role, as a teacher, then take some time understand your role's function and how it differs from instructing a set of yoga poses. Once you're clear, you'll know better the pathway that you will take in your ongoing development and where you'll want to focus your time toward continued study.

So why is it even relevant to include a lesson on this topic. Well, I had a conversation with a friend who isn't a yoga teacher, and she questioned me on the difference between a yoga teacher and yoga instructor. You see, my friend does practice yoga, and our conversation really revolved around her desire to find a space where she could plug in and create consistency in her practice. She mentioned that when she was looking on particular studio websites that she saw the word "instructors" listed rather than "teachers."

She expressed that she wasn't seeking someone to just "instruct" her, or lead her through a set of the yoga poses; she desired to be led by someone who could teach, impart knowledge, and apply wisdom that goes beyond the physicality of the asana. My friend and yoga student feels like there is a difference between these terms, and because of this conversation, I felt there is great relevance and value for yoga teachers to explore this further and to ultimately choose what type of teacher — or instructor — you desire to be. So essentially, it does matter.

## Reflective Exercise

Journal your approach and what type of teacher you desire to be. How will you take action from this desired approach?

LESSON 7:

# Meet Students Where They Are

---

"Meet students where they are, not where you want
them to be."

— DR. MARA LEE GRAYSON

It's easy to focus on preparing the poses and sequences you will teach and forget about the various people you will encounter as you teach a yoga class. If you aren't careful, you'll begin to see the yoga poses rather than the people in your classes. In this lesson, learn the technique of how to release attachment to a desire planned sequence in order to identify and meet the needs of the students who are actually right in front of you and meet them where they are within their unique practice experience. Learn three key sequencing principles that will support your ability to provide structure in your classes while developing spontaneity to adapt and adjust your planned sequence according to the students in your class.

The origins of yoga date back some five thousand years ago, and the classical yoga asanas take us back to the ancient yogic texts in the Hatha Yoga Pradipika. So it's safe to say that you may have the skill to introduce asana in an interesting, creative way through sequencing while remaining effective by focusing on simplicity rather than making class sequences overly complex.

In this lesson, I am going to share with you three principles for keeping your class sequences simple, yet impactful, and in congruency with what I believe the concentrated sustained flow state of yoga was intended and designed to offer the practitioner. I have had quite a few conversations and mentoring sessions with teachers who express concern that students might get bored if they do not continually create new and fresh sequences. Yoga teachers often take on an overwhelming pressure to constantly keep their sequence plans highly creative and sometimes overly complex in an effort to entertain students. It's almost this cycle of reinventing the wheel, and this approach will eventually wear on you and exhaust your preparation process for teaching.

Let's explore three highly effective principles you can incorporate into your sequence planning that support simplicity while lessening the stress of getting caught up in the never-ending wheel of creating new sequences.

## Develop Mastery of the Mini-Sequence

During your yoga teacher training, you are taught a framework or foundational structure for sequencing yoga classes. From this foundational structured sequence plan, you will begin to incorporate mini-sequences within the category of each of the various sequencing collections of yoga postures as they apply to the element of action and intention they exhibit. Mini-sequences consist of a max of three to four yoga postures practiced symmetrically, so on each side. That's it. The more yoga postures you try to link together increases a greater opportunity for you, the teacher, to get caught up mentally trying to remember your sequence. When you try to link too many postures together, you also heighten the risk of students losing stability, which increases the potential opportunity of injury that results from fatiguing one side of the body more than the other.

Mini-sequences are a collection of organized postures with familiarity in alignment and action principles. They also comprise the various qualities or segments found within pieces of the yoga class. For example, you would have a mini-sequence for the opening, warmup phase of class, the strength building, and balance segment all the way to the end of the class. Mastery of mini-sequences allows you to place and fit them together as you would fit a piece into a puzzle, to create the overall picture of the class experience. The mini-sequence approach simplifies sequencing and makes class preparation seem less overwhelming when you think about organizing enough sequences within say a sixty-minute time frame.

The mini-sequences are thoughtfully and skillfully put together in your structured plan, and the mastery part of the mini-sequence approach shows up when you spend time, in repetition, practicing the sequences first for yourself. Teaching the mini-sequence over and over until you've mastered the ability to lead others through it will help you feel the confidence to move on to create a new mini-sequence that you will then add in the next principle that I want to share.

## 90/10 Rule

The second principle of applying simplicity to sequencing is the 90/10 Rule. Once you have mastered your collection of mini-sequences, it is time to put these mini-sequences together to form the bigger picture of the entire yoga class. This is where you begin to create sequence plans that consist of ninety percent of the "go-to" mini-sequences you have mastered.

This approach supports your ability to step into classes with a structured planned sequence but also allows room for spontaneity because, in order to become a highly effective teacher, you will need to know how to adjust and adapt your overall sequencing plan quickly. Just because you planned out a sequence for that given day doesn't mean that the student you planned for is the one that actually shows up to the class. It is important to develop a teaching methodology and approach that supports the balance of structure and spontaneity.

What about the ten-percent aspect of the 90/10 Rule? This applies to the amount of class time you designate to teaching something new or sharing a particular emphasis for that class. This could be a new transition, new mini-sequence, or new point of focus and emphasis that you will be sharing throughout the practice experience. In order to remain effective and confident within your teaching, I highly encourage you to let only ten percent of your overall class time account for the teaching or sharing of a new focus or emphasis. Within the ten percent of time you are growing as a teacher because this is the space where you are teaching what you need to learn at the same time.

This small yet powerful percentage of your class makes learning and implementing new information more accessible for you as a teacher to share rather than becoming overwhelmed with how you might begin adding new information or knowledge you are acquiring through your ongoing pursuits of study. Ten percent is manageable and highly effective when it comes to adding something new to your sequencing plan.

The 90/10 Rule also offers you the opportunity to enhance your capacity to step into the classroom with a plan and then actually empty yourself of any attachment to a set plan. Within this approach, you can show up fully present, aware, and ready to meet the needs of the students that are right in front of you, in the real time act of teaching. Applying these principles within your sequencing will offer to you a huge developmental opportunity as a teacher. More importantly, this will allow for you, as the teacher, to fade into the background of the class experience and let the teachings of yoga be showcased. Yoga becomes highly accessible when teachers are thoughtful and considerate within their approach to sequencing in this regard.

I also want to share with you what happens when you reverse the 90/10 Rule. This shows up when teachers choose to create overly complex sequences. Rather than ninety percent of the class sequence being your go-to mini-sequences, ninety percent is devoted to the creation of a collection of asana sequences that have yet to be explored or level of mastery achieved in the experience. They have resided within the construct of the mind, and they have often not yet been given ample time to explore and practice them. I'm speaking from experience here. I have encountered this approach first-hand, and it is not an approach I would want to keep using. When we reverse the 90/10 approach to sequencing, we get too caught up in the mental space of remembering because, quite honestly, if we've never really spent a lot of time seeking to understand the new concept or new sequence, there isn't a familiarity when it comes to remembering.

## Repetition

Repetition shows up for you as the teacher in the first principle of mastering the mini-sequence, and now I want to highlight this aspect in regard to the impact that repetition can have on student's ability to access the residual impact of the practice of yoga. Early in my development as a yoga teacher,

I began to deepen my understanding of repetition within the learning process. I discovered that repetition is a key learning aid because it helps transition a skill from the conscious to the subconscious. Through repetition, a skill is practiced and rehearsed over time, and it gradually becomes easier, accessible, and more memorable. This is where the concept of reminding students until they remember becomes an important attribute in effective and impactful teaching. Repetition supports remembrance.

I'll add here the importance of educating ourselves on the intelligence and biomechanics of the body's ability to move. Movement is not a one-size-fits-all approach. It is important to have an overall broad stroke of understanding of the various movements of the body. It's a start point. For movement-based teachers, it makes sense to devote time in deeper study of understanding how to equip others to move with efficiency and acknowledge the natural intuitive intelligence within the function and movements of our bodies.

When it comes to the principle of repetition, we do need to be mindful that we are moving our bodies in a variety of ways and on a variety of planes. This will speak to the styles of yoga that only teach a set sequence without any varying movements. As a student, if we only practice this one set style repetitively, then eventually, our bodies will remember the movements, and yes, even yoga carries a heightened risk of injury when we only move the body one way repetitively. So set-sequence asana practiced in a repetitious manner consistency can wear and tear on the body. This is where cross-training within various styles of yoga is an important element within the practice. Exploring various styles and movement practices will decrease potential overuse injuries when we become comfortable within a known pattern of movement.

The body is so brilliant in its intelligence, and because of the learning possibilities that come with repetition, the body will certainly adapt to the positions or movements that we place it in. We are creatures of habit, so repetition brings comfort and familiarity, as well. Take note of the mental tendencies that can creep in and distract you while applying this principle to sequencing and practicing yoga. This will happen for the students you lead. Within the concept of simplicity of sequencing and repetition, we also want to be mindful that we are offering students a variety of movement patterns and ways that we approach transitioning in and out of postures. This doesn't mean our sequencing needs to be overly complex, but we do need to offer varying ways within the simplicity and principles I've already shared. This is a great place for the 90/10 Rule. You can teach the same mini-sequences repetitively yet add in variety within the ten percent portion.

## SPACED REPETITION

Another important aspect of repetition to highlight here is the interval at which a skill is repeated. Spaced repetition is a learning technique that incorporates increasing intervals of time between the practice of previously learned sequences. Applying this within the approach to the Vinyasa style of yoga, there is the component of tempo that is present within the rhythm and flow of this class style. Tempo affords you a great opportunity to vary the class emphasis in accordance with the length of holds and the moments of pause that you can sprinkle in to impact the class experience. You have the ability to vary the tempo of the class, which gives students yet another way to create a unique and different encounter in the practice experience and invites the curious evaluation that comes within the interacting of the postures as they are held longer or when students are invited to move with a steadiness and stability when the tempo and pace becomes quicker.

You can use the principle of repetition and tempo within other styles of yoga you might teach. This doesn't apply solely to Vinyasa or flow-style classes, although, I would highly encourage you to pay close attention to this concept if you do teach the Vinyasa style. You can certainly add all of these key principles of sequencing with simplicity within a variety of styles you might teach, even the Yin and Restorative styles of yoga have elements of all of these approaches that support simplicity before complexity within the asana sequencing.

## Simplicity and Balance

I'll now tie all of this together within the overall understanding of simplicity. How do these three principles help to keep sequencing simple? Why does simplicity offer students an opportunity to allow the practice and teachings of yoga to make an impact on their lives?

Once you are clear on your intention that supports simplicity, your next evaluation in class planning is to look through the lens of balance. Keep in mind that within Hatha Yoga, the word ha–tha refers to a union of polarities—in other words, balance. Regarding this balance of polarities, if your desire is to activate and encourage an active approach within the practice you're teaching, you can find the right balance of strong postures to ignite organization and muscular activation within your students' experience. At the same time, you can offer them reflective moments of stillness sprinkled throughout so that they can sense the sustainable effort and the balance of ease.

Your approach toward simplicity helps support the creation

of balance. Within all things in life, balance is a necessary state for our overall well-being. We can see balance played out in a variety of aspects in our lives. When you choose simplicity in your sequencing approach, you also choose balance and intention. Simplicity doesn't mean easy. It's more about accessibility and an opportunity for the practice to become clearer for the students you lead. It provides great clarity for you as a teacher, as well.

Complexity isn't bad, and there are times when sequencing can have a flavor of complexity as long as you remain aligned in the thoughtfulness of your communication, guidance and support of students as you move them within the complexity of the various shapes and transitional movements. Complexity has its place, but use great discernment to evaluate your intent and agenda for offering a more complex sequence. My desire is that you are equipped with methods and principles that support discernment and eliminate distractions of feeling like overly complex and challenging asana sequences are a necessity in order to entice or entertain students and keep them coming back to class.

Approaching sequencing within simplicity offers you a wonderful and intentionally organized way to incorporate a layered learning experience in your classroom. If you have the opportunity to teach more than one class a week, then use these class times to master the simplicity of the sequences your offer by repeating the sequences, while also infusing the ten percent. This could be the chance for students to encounter the same poses and sequences from a new lens and deeper understanding of analyzing how they are being within the action of creating the yoga pose shape.

If you're thinking the students may get bored with your class if you aren't teaching a new sequence each and every class, turn those ideas into an approach that allows you to expand and deepen the learning experience. Take a simple sequence and add the creativity found within the layers that go beyond and below the surface of the experience, always needing to be filled with new sequences. Get creative by using these three principles that offer success to your students and to you as a teacher.

Simplicity invites students to learn and loosen the grip of limitations or expectations they've placed upon themselves. Simplicity creates a learning space that also lessens frustration and chances for miscommunication. When sequencing is too complex, it diminishes the space of learning and heightens moments of disconnect. Too much complexity will also increase the cues you will have to use to guide students into unfamiliar territory, which increases the chance of miscommunication. If it's hard for you to say or cue, then it's going to be hard for students to receive and understand where you're trying to lead them. Too much complexity can interrupt the opportunity to reflect and choose the most appropriate responses while moving in and out of postures.

I'll close out this lesson with a quote by Aristotle regarding the importance of repetition in education: "It is frequent repetition that produces a natural tendency." When it comes to being a yoga teacher, you are an educator. Your role as teacher is to equip students with the best opportunity for learning, developing, and expanding their understanding of who they are and why they do what they do on the yoga mat and out in their lives. It's through the facilitation of a yoga asana class that most of us are teaching and guiding others, so it only makes sense that we devote ourselves to understanding the best approach toward making this learning opportunity available and accessible for the students we lead. Simplicity supports this model and approach, where complexity has tendencies to complicate and hinder learning. Keep it simple.

## Reflective Exercise

What will be your approach to sequencing? Write out your sequencing framework and evaluate how you will apply simplicity within the three key principles from this lesson into your overall approach to sequencing.

# Teaching Yoga in Various Locations

"Never doubt that a small group of thoughtful,
committed citizens can change the world; indeed, it's
the only thing that ever has."
— MARGARET MEAD

To meet students where they are, you'll need to understand and evaluate the setting and location in which you teach. Various locations may present different challenges and require alternative methods and approaches toward teaching the practice of yoga. In this lesson, learn specific ways to prepare and teach yoga in nontraditional settings outside of a yoga studio. I would say that seeking to meet people where they are in life and within and along their yoga practice journey ranks highly in my overall desire to develop and grow as a yoga teacher.

This is also my approach in all other aspects of my life. We spend a lot of time in yoga teacher trainings, studying and learning through a more left-brained focus. We read books, we write papers and journal, and we practice the technical skill set aspect of teaching. These are all important attributes to work on and skills to develop as a teacher, but you must also consider the relational right-brain aspect of teaching. Paying attention to the development of this aspect will ultimately equip and impact the overall experience you have as you develop and grow as a yoga teacher.

We often hear that yoga is for everyone, and yes, it is, but I also believe that the element of timing is involved, as well.

Everyone will not fall in love with the practice in the same timing that someone else might have. For some, they may not be ready to commit to what the practice might ask or require of them. Some will be curious but not curious enough yet to continue the pursuit of exploring and learning more. Some, though, will immediately dive into the pursuit and quest. So, how do you develop and teach in a way that meets the needs of the variety of students you will encounter?

Yoga class is probably one of the few gatherings that truly provides a landscape for discovery where a diverse group of individuals converges with a vast array of intentions, attributes, and expectations that they bring into the practice space with them. I think of the yoga class as a setting where you will find the chakras on display and within the variety of humanity that shows up on that given day. There's that aspect of timing coming in again.

If you're going to devote yourself to meeting the needs of this vast array of humanity, that will be represented in the classes you lead, then it will be important to develop the relational aspect of your role as teacher. Understanding and discerning how to share the practice in relevant ways that meets this vast spectrum of individuals where they are in that given practice experience is a skill worth developing.

For you to find depth and longevity as a yoga teacher, I encourage you to seek out teaching opportunities that aren't necessarily found within the traditional setting we might think of when we pursue teacher training. We know that the benefits of practicing yoga provides a system for managing and eliminating the suffering that the habits of our minds bring to us in the life. If yoga is for everyone, then as a yoga teacher, it is important that you become versed in accessing and adapting the practice to meet the needs of the ones you are sharing the practice with.

The best way to begin developing this aspect of your relational teaching skill set is to think of the practice from the viewpoint of relevance then make a list of the top three benefits of practicing yoga. Next, evaluate the setting you are teaching in. How can you incorporate the teachings of yoga, along with the benefits, and offer an experience that is relevant to the individuals you are teaching and within the setting you are teaching in? You get creative and adapt the teachings and benefits of yoga to meet the needs of the particular student you're teaching while sparking curiosity that begins to plant a seed within the individuals you're teaching.

That seed might not take root right away, and it may be a season of time before the curiosity is sparked to discover and uncover more, but that is not your responsibility. Your role and responsibility is not to make everyone fall in love with yoga and become a dedicated practitioner in an instant. Your role is to provide an experience that offers yoga in a way that is relevant and meets the needs of the collective you're teaching that given day and in that given time. It's like how we approach our personal practice. We show up and dedicate ourselves to the practice of being present for the experience, then, when the practice is over, we step back and take our hands off any perceived result. Rather, we trust in the commitment that we made and that in time, and with practice, we will remember and experience the fullness of the present moment again.

Oftentimes, we hear that for some people wanting to try yoga, the hardest part is actually going to a class. Once people walk into the yoga practice space, then it's our responsibility, as yoga teachers, to move toward these individuals, to be approachable and real. Just because you become a yoga teacher doesn't make you any more "advanced" or above the students you teach. If you get swept up in that mindset, then the ego has crept in, and you will not develop the relational aspect of teaching that I have mentioned. In fact, you could become a barrier or distraction for students and diminish their ability to create and develop an autonomous practice experience due to the shift of the practice seeming more like a performance-driven system rather than a practice of presence and the elimination of the habitual suffering our minds create.

The best way to expand and develop the breadth of your teaching skill set is to teach in a variety of locations and not limiting yourself to the locations that are most obvious, such as the yoga studio setting. As you teach in locations such as gyms and fitness centers or outdoor recreational venues, you will begin to release attachments that would suggest that the practice must look a certain way or the setting must be set in a way for students to be successful. Setting the tone and emphasis is important, but it's important to be mindful and remember that your role isn't to create an experience that students attach to that would suggest that certain features, such as the temperature of the room or the lights and sounds must be just right in order for them to have a successful experience. Rather, the success comes within the facilitation of an experience where students are guided beyond the exterior of doing and into the interior of reflective evaluation and deeper understanding of how they are moving not only on their mats but within their relationships to life off the mat.

Whether you teach in a studio or a fitness center, or to a collection of high school students, the intention is the same. How can you show up and hold space for these individuals to move safely within their bodies while experiencing the balance of stillness at the same time? How can we, as teachers, share the practice in a way that invites others to explore? We want to make a serious acknowledgment without taking ourselves too seriously or making the practice another rigidity in life, another box to check. How can we, as teachers, guide and lead in a way that provides the relevance that the yoga practice is more than something we do if we have time but rather all other aspects fall into place around the dedicated time we devote to remaining consistent to practicing? This is an ongoing pursuit.

When we teach in a variety of settings, to a variety of students, within a variety of ages and accessibility, we begin to discern and teach in a way that meets people where they are. We give the gift of knowing that the practice doesn't have to look a certain way and that it can be adapted and adjusted to meet their needs.

Ultimately, we teach what we deem important. Take some time to evaluate what you consider important within the practice and what you would want others to glean and learn from the experience and practice of yoga. You might even find that all of the extras you thought you needed to focus more heavily upon—the lighting, the perfect playlist, and the lavender-scented cloths—are not the focal point of the practice experience. Perhaps the beautiful collective of individuals coming together to share a relational experience where connection is experienced deserves more of our focus and attention.

## Reflective Exercise

Make notes on how you might need to adjust and adapt your approach to teaching yoga within various settings such as outdoors, gyms, fitness centers, senior centers, or high schools. Evaluate what other nontraditional settings might be available for you to share the practice of yoga in your community.

# PART TWO:

# Confidence

# Introduction

Merriam-Webster defines confidence as "faith or belief that one will act in a right, proper, or effective way." Confidence prepares us to move forward and pursue opportunities while encouraging others to do the same. Confidence also supports us in recognizing our capacity to remember and try again.

As you begin to develop and grow within your role as a yoga teacher, you build upon the foundation laid in your teaching training and real-time teaching experiences. The ability to sustain the work of service teaching yoga presents itself in a variety of ways. A key aspect of this representation comes within the invisible realm of confidence that begins to form and support the ongoing development and enduring effort that teaching a life practice such as yoga requires. Within this invisible realm, the quiet acknowledgement of our capacity to sustain this endeavor emerges. As you begin to remind students of their capacity to move with efficiency and skill, you also equip yourself with the same assurance.

Through the dedicated effort of showing up not only for the students you teach, but also for yourself as a teacher, you can begin to sense a space of deep understanding within — a space that becomes more familiar. As genuine confidence emerges, it is felt, and others come to trust more deeply in their own capacity to know this space for themselves. In this section, we will dig deeper into the qualities of building confidence as a yoga teacher.

# Doubting Your Identity

"Be you. You are sacred."
— LAILAH GIFTY AKITA

Look to other yoga teachers for inspiration and encouragement, but take note that your teaching pathway is uniquely yours, for you to develop and share. In this lesson, we'll explore how you identify with being a yoga teacher, what that looks like and how this impacts your effectiveness teaching yoga.

When it comes to identifying with a particular aspect of yourself and your pursuits, how do you currently identify as a yoga teacher? What does that look like for you? We hear often, and especially within marketing efforts for yoga teacher training programs, about becoming a yoga teacher. That's an interesting statement because it almost sets someone up from the very beginning to become disappointed or disillusioned that a short period of six months, or possibly a thirty-day-immersive experience, will instantly or magically turn you into a yoga teacher. It just isn't that easy. What I have found to be true is that it's anything but that.

Yoga teacher training is a necessary start point, but when the training is over, you will have to continue to learn, apply, evaluate, and dedicate to the ongoing pursuit of being a yoga teacher. How long does it take to become or be a yoga teacher? Well, I don't have the answer to that question, but I can say that after more than twenty years, I've yet to fully arrive.

I'm a little farther along the path, and my understanding now of my role, my identity, as a yoga teacher is nothing like the one I identified with two decades ago. In fact, when I decided to seek training to teach, it was merely because I enjoyed the practice and saw it as a path to generating a little income to support my family while doing and sharing what I enjoyed with others. That was my motivation. Yoga had captured my attention, and from what I shared in the introduction to this book, yoga arrived at a pivotal time in my life.

Although the identifying marker of motivation has changed, I do still enjoy the practice and love sharing it with others. My quest has become the ongoing pursuit to understand the practice more fully for myself first, and from that deeper personal understanding, I might share and support the development of other teachers as we collectively serve our communities teaching yoga.

## Identity Marker

As we explore identity further, let's first look at what aspects, or markers, support the defining of identity. Within the context of being a yoga teacher, what markers would you say support your identity: challenging and creative sequencing, the extras that you provide in the class experience, or the carefully curated playlist? How would you identify with being a yoga teacher if you weren't actively teaching asana? I recently dove into this aspect with a mentorship client, and it has really stood out to me as a topic that deserves deeper exploration. Does your identity shift and change according to the marker of whether or not you are actively teaching asana classes?

Understanding your identity and the markers you use in identifying with your role as a yoga teacher will help to bring clarity to what being a yoga teacher means and exemplifies for you. This clarity will further support you within the various seasons of your teaching journey. When you question your identity, it is important to make sure you aren't attaching certain elements or stipulations within the markers that you use to identify yourself as a teacher. The markers you use 1) may not be true and 2) might be lacking in the full scope of who you really are within that role and identity as a yoga teacher. When you understand the concept of seasons and how change is a big determining factor in that assessment, then you'll begin to loosen the attachments that place your identity reliant solely upon the action, or inaction, that you perceive is taking place in which you fulfill your identity.

In the beginning of my teaching career, I totally based my identity upon the marker of how well I could lead others through a set of yoga poses. Honestly, at that time in my practice and development as a new teacher, it was all about the yoga pose. But, then again, why wouldn't it be? That is the start point for most of us. It's what captures our attention in the beginning. The asana is the physical manifestation of what we associate with yoga when, interestingly, the "yoga" is actually the residue of experience that one encounters through the initiation or integration of all aspects and pieces of the practice. Asana is just one piece, one limb, of the practice. In the beginning, for me, the quest to become a yoga teacher revolved around the marker of asana. It's an important element, but it isn't the sole element when it comes to identifying with the yoga practice.

## Consumed with Creativity

Caught up in creativity. Is this you? I love creative sequencing, but there must be a thoughtful intelligence present that backs the creative element. If you're not careful, your identifying marker as a yoga teacher could begin to revolve so heavily around creative sequencing that you become consumed with creativity to the extent that the impact falls flat because the teaching doesn't back the sequencing approach. Creativity can consume you in your preparation, and the layers of the other aspects of teaching yoga can fall behind or become nonexistent. When we are more heavily focused on the creation of class sequences, consumed with creativity and possibly complexity, then we miss the big picture that the role of asana plays within the overall practice experience of yoga. It's sneaky. If you aren't careful, you can quickly allow your identity to become consumed with this aspect. Rather, could you use asana creatively as a vehicle to explore the deeper, yet subtle, layers of the practice experience?

When we study the ancient texts of yoga and, in particular, the yoga sutra and the path that Patanjali lays out for the practice of yoga, asana constitutes a limb of the practice. Yet how much of the Sutras are devoted to the importance of creative sequencing of the asana? None. In fact, Patanjali chooses, instead, to describe the limb of asana within the context of exploring a way of being rather than the quest or act of doing. Asana, as described in the texts, is the seat. It is the seat we take that prepares the body for stillness. So the asana is the beautiful paradox of moving toward stillness.

I found this true for myself. There is power to be found in preparing the body for the experience of stillness and the inner experience of solitude. Asana is definitely a catalyst for this profound experience. I will also add here that my identity and understanding of this piece, this limb, has evolved and changed with my experiences practicing yoga. I have found that an important skill set for a yoga teacher to develop is one that continually seeks to understand and meet people where they are in the practice experience. Because of the evolving experiences I have witnessed in my own practice, I am better equipped to hold the same space for others, knowing that like me, others might be identifying with the yoga practice more through the reflection of asana while others begin to explore different aspects of the practice that are beyond the physicality.

When we remain consumed with creative sequencing, we just might be teaching others that this is the sole aspect of practicing yoga. What then, when the changes of life are encountered, including changes in physical abilities, will students identify with within the practice of yoga? Asanas are designed for us to use as tools to excavate and dig deeper into the soil of the practice experience not to merely till up the soil on the surface. If creative sequencing is the sole marker of our identity as a yoga teacher then we — and the students we teach — will remain on the surface.

Through the discipline of identifying with asana as a powerful seat within the vehicle of discovery, my identity has adapted to support others by seeking ways to lead students in assessing their own experience and identity in the practice. This guidance invites students to submerge themselves below the surface of what is seen or represented within the concept of yoga through the yoga poses. Sequencing is very important, and I am a huge advocate for teachers to understand and develop the skills to lead others successfully through the yoga asana practice.

When you find yourself consumed with the pursuit of creativity and constantly seek to use asana sequences as a means of keeping students entertained or engaged, then you have begun to identify yoga with the pose rather the residual experience that has the power to offer transformative action in our lives. This perspective is signaling to you that you are attaching your identity as a yoga teacher within a perspective that is actually skewing your deeper purpose as a teacher. Your purpose as a teacher is not to be known solely for your creative choreographed sequence; that is the ego. Your purpose is to lead other skillfully, using the linking of asana in a way that meets their needs and supports a deeper understanding of themselves through the practice of yoga. When the source of your identity is consumed with creative sequencing, then you most likely are going to find that you really aren't creating a student-centered class experience that supports the needs of the actual students who show up for class. You are creating the sequence for yourself.

## Disappointment

I had a conversation with another teacher, and she expressed to me her disappointment when she has planned out her class sequence—let me emphasize the words "her sequence" in this—and the students who show up for the class are not the ones she prepared for. What I perceived from this conversation is that she is basically planning her class sequences for herself, not for the students.

It's important to understand that the skill sets of practicing yoga and teaching yoga are totally different. I have come to learn that just because I practice a certain style, or even a certain posture, that doesn't mean it translates naturally into the sequences I will lead others through. Just because it serves my personal practice does not mean that it serves others or that I need to teach it.

I do believe, and know to be true for myself, that my time on the mat in my personal practice does contribute and inspire my teaching. My personal practice time is a vital aspect in the development of my effectiveness as a teacher. Knowing the practice for yourself first will support your ability to lead someone else through their journey of development within their practice experience. Students aren't seeking for you to come in and perform all your knowledge for them. They are more interested in the authentic relational aspect that you bring to the practice experience as you lead them through a created experience that you actually know because you have been there before. Teaching becomes much fuller and sustainable when you teach from the place that you know rather than trying to replicate an experience from memorization or delivery of an analytical, left-brained approach to a practice experience that is much more than that aspect of our being.

As teachers, we facilitate a learning space that is creative in nature. We partner with students in a collaborative effort to create an experience in the setting of the yoga class that supports the collective and at the same time the individual autonomous encounter taking place as each individual begins to identify and relate to their unique practice experience. It's actually a beautiful paradox. Each student is given the opportunity to be in a cohesive group experience, while at the same time, invited to enjoy their own personal encounter within the practice that given day. I just love this aspect of teaching.

Within the context of disappointment, it's important to evaluate your approach and desire to teach. Could you subconsciously desire for students to encounter the yoga practice the way you prefer to experience it? Do you get disappointed when you aren't able to deliver the sequence you had planned? It's helpful to note that if you do find yourself in the space of disappointment over not being able to teach the sequence that you had planned, to take some time reflecting back again upon your identity, purpose, and role as a yoga teacher. Ask yourself, "What is my agenda?" Are you attached to your sequence plan in a way that keeps you from actually seeing the students you are leading? Could you be misguided about the role and purpose that asana plays within the practice experience?

As a yoga teacher, you have a choice. If your emphasis and focus resides primarily upon the asana and the execution of your planned sequence then that is the meaning and emphasis that students will translate and apply to their own understanding of the practice. This is what you will teach students. If you are the only teacher that a student ever has then you will be limiting their opportunity of discovering the depths and fullness of the entire eight-limb path to be explored within the yoga practice.

## Lack of Clear Direction

Developing a clear point of view and direction as a teacher requires a willingness to pursue the work of an internal investigation of a better understanding of your personal relationship with the practice of yoga. From this understanding, you will discern the direction that aligns with your distinct purpose, but you will have to spend time getting clear on what that is first.

Your personal practice time will become a deciding factor in the ability to discern and gather clarity on your aligned purpose as a teacher. Dedicating time to the ongoing pursuit of being a student of the practice will contribute toward your ability to pick up on the innate calling that you sensed when you began your journey toward becoming a yoga teacher. Although wonderful and definitely a contributor, simply loving the practice of yoga and accumulating knowledge and training will not develop you fully into an effective yoga teacher. Dedication is required in becoming still while attuning to the deep level of discernment and promptings in order to assess this clear direction. I often advise anyone who is on a quest for clarity to get still. Get still and sit with whatever you are seeking, whether clarity and guidance or the ability to discern within an important decision that is being asked of you. Be still and know.

Lastly, if you desire to sustain and create longevity within the service of teaching yoga, then an ongoing commitment to examination, re-examination even, will become necessary as you pursue this great work. If you avoid this dedicated time, then you will most likely find yourself looking out at what other teachers are pursuing and begin seeking to replicate their path. Learning and gleaning from other yoga teachers is a great motivation as long as it doesn't begin to take the place of the work you spend dedicated to your own understanding of your clear direction and teaching path. Over the past two decades, I have explored various teaching opportunities, ones that have challenged me to grow and ones that have supported me in developing the skills I desire to develop in my effectiveness as a teacher. I have had seasons where I needed to re-evaluate where I was and the direction I was headed in. From this evaluation, I have changed course in order to align back into my purpose and calling as a teacher. Just as the flow of life and circumstances are in flux and change is present, the pursuit you take as a teacher will also shift and change.

To support this flux with more ease, your time in solitude and reflection will support this ongoing ability to adapt and adjust within the various seasons of your teaching career. This time will also support your ability to trust in your role and identity as a yoga teacher and to understand that it's about you, but then again it really isn't. You are a facilitator. You share and allow the teachings of yoga to pass through you, not from you. My personal desire for ongoing development as a yoga teacher, and the desire I have for you, as well, is that you devote the necessary time needed in the pursuit of knowing the practice of yoga more fully for yourself, first and foremost. From that deeper understanding, the ongoing pursuit becomes the bigger work of seeking to not disrupt the flow of the teachings that will pass though you so that the teachings might be encountered more fully by those you lead. This development supports the great opportunity of leadership which we will explore in the next section of this book.

## Reflective Exercise

Evaluate how much time you spend scrolling through social media to see what other teachers are doing. When you feel yourself pulled into comparison, stop and write it down. Begin to notice what markers you are identifying with. Take note of any feelings of doubt or comparison and seek to rewire your thoughts to affirm your unique gift and identity as a yoga teacher.

# Collaboration over Competition

"Collaboration allows us to know more than we are capable of knowing ourselves."

— PAUL SOLARZ

There is enough yoga to go around, and there is no room for competition within the action of service. In this lesson, discover how you can build healthy relationships and collaborations with other teachers that will support deeper learning through collaborative teaching experiences.

I would like to think that competition and comparison wouldn't be a pitfall found within the yoga industry and, in particular, among fellow yoga teachers, but realistically, that's not the case. Yoga teachers are not immune to the plight of the human condition, the ego, and the habit of measuring ourselves and our pursuits against those of others. But why do we find ourselves easily distracted at times or looking outside ourselves?

Let's explore all of this, and by the end of this lesson, you will be equipped with six distinct areas of focus that will support you in avoiding the pitfall of the comparison trap. I will also share how to notice when you've fallen into the trap of competition and comparison, and I will offer some tangible ways to get out of the trap and realign yourself into the bigger work of serving your community by teaching yoga.

## Trap of Comparison

How do you know when you have been entrapped by comparison? From my experience, it begins when you find yourself looking out rather than looking within. You spend more time focusing on what others are doing and begin questioning what you are doing. Then uncertainty creeps in. As students of the practice of yoga, we come to find out quickly that the practice is very much a journey inward. The practice is an introspective pursuit. It becomes a quest to discover and know ourselves more deeply, and in order to do so, we begin to evaluate why we do what we do.

For most of us, the pursuit begins as we move our bodies in and out of a variety of shapes we call yoga poses. These shapes soon become the vehicles that will take us on this journey inward. Since the physicality of the asana is very much seen and reflected within community yoga class settings, we can quickly find ourselves consumed with the exterior of the experience. The practice of yoga will remain on the surface of what is seen outwardly unless we are guided to choose to explore the depths of the interior, internal experience that awaits anyone who practices yoga. It becomes an inquiry of how we are being versus solely what we are doing. I have often wondered why we say that we are "doing" yoga. Isn't the "yoga" experienced as the residue around the nature of our being that is less about producing action and more about cultivating a new way of being?

For practitioners of yoga, there is not magic understanding or timing as to when this deeper revelation might be discovered. As a student, we are presented with the decision and discernment to seek out guidance and deeper understanding of the teachings of yoga. And in that seeking, we will either find teachers who teach us how and guide us toward this interior encounter within the practice, or we encounter teachers, or instructors, whose focus remains primarily on the exterior of the practice experience. This is where, as a yoga teacher, you are presented with a powerful question of inquiry: what kind of teacher will you be? This clarity will become an important contributor when it comes to evaluating comparison and competition along your teaching path.

If you choose to stay on the exterior, looking outside of yourself to try to replicate another teacher's experience, then you will miss the unique opportunity you have to make an impact teaching yoga. There is only one you. I encourage you to always be true to yourself and your unique gift of sharing and teaching yoga. Be inspired and encouraged by other teachers, but remain faithful and dedicated to your path of service. There are several points to consider for getting clear about what kind of teacher you desire to be and the commitment you then make to grow and develop within that chosen space.

## Understanding Comparison

There is a healthy approach to understanding comparison so that it will serve to benefit you rather than keeping you stuck in the muck and mire of the hustle of keeping up with the endeavors of other teachers. The landscape of yoga studios, gyms, and any other spaces where we interact regularly with other teachers would benefit greatly by instilling and implementing healthy interactions among the teaching staff.

Comparison is a fundamental human impulse. Within this fundamental aspect, comparison also has the potential to become a great motivator. It's tricky, though. You'll want to sharpen your awareness to when you become out of balance within this relationship. In other words, you must be mindful to when comparison becomes unhealthy. Noticing the direction that the motivation of comparison has and where it leads you is of great importance. If left unattended, or unevaluated, you could possibly find yourself headed in the wrong direction or misaligned with your unique call and path as a teacher.

If we spend time affirming this thought, then the actions that will come from this thought stream will be those that reside in abundance and knowing. Knowing that you do not have to compete or look outside of yourself to see if you measure up with another teacher. You will also diminish the distraction of doubt that will creep in and veer you off your unique teaching path.

When you are clear on who you are and what type of teacher you desire to be, then your actions will align with that thought pattern. Then you'll find yourself moving along the path that supports your desired development as a teacher rather than finding yourself on a path of impersonating another teacher.

## What is comparison?

In order to understand comparison better, it's important to first understand the behavior so that you can then redirect your thoughts. As mentioned, that will ultimately affect the actions you take or don't take. There is a cyclical cause and effect within comparison. Researchers use the term comparison-targets when noticing the behavioral qualities we most closely identify with, as well as, those within our personal sphere of influence. The evaluations we relate to most significantly — appearance, relationships, wealth, professional achievement, or even goals — become even more specific within our comparison targets. We begin to make or use comparisons targets as a way of evaluating ourselves. With this evaluation, there are effects of upward and downward comparisons, which are dependent upon how we process the information we receive when we make self-evaluating comparisons with others. I'll speak to this further in just a moment.

## Six Focal Points for Avoiding the Comparison Trap

### COUNT YOUR BLESSINGS

First things first, cultivate a mindset of gratitude. This sounds simple, yet if you think of your mindset as a garden, then in order to cultivate a garden that supports growth and vibrancy, it will need to be tended to well. Trying to grow a garden or anything requires effort—sometimes a lot of effort even. It requires attention and a directed focus toward the goal of healthy growth and development of that which we're desiring to plant.

I don't have a vegetable garden, but I do like to have seasonal plants and flowers around my home. Once planted, I cannot merely sit back and think that they will take care of themselves. Instead, I must remind myself—and sometimes enlist others—to nurture and take care of them. Our mindset is the same way. If we are to cultivate a mindset that avoids unhealthy comparisons and instead plant seeds of gratitude and acknowledgment of our blessings, we must also be willing to be patient and consistent. As we focus our attention toward the growth of gratitude and blessings within our mindset, then we will find there is no room for the unhealthy weeds of comparison and negative competition within the garden of our mind.

For the most part, individuals have the capacity of gratitude. Like yoga, gratitude is a conscious practice. Our minds are tricky, and if left without concern or application of an "attitude of gratitude," the mind will quickly take us down the trail of despair and suffering.

In regard to social media and the status and importance we place on these platforms, we need to evaluate the time spent there. Are you cultivating real encounters and then nurturing those who have invested in you as a follower? Or are you continually seeking more followers? The amount of time you actually spend nurturing the followers you currently have will be an indicator of how much emphasis you will place in the aspect of nourishing and growing relationships when you gain more. This also applies to your business email list. It doesn't matter how many new contacts you gain if you aren't nurturing the ones you already have. When we talk of gratitude for what we have, let's also reflect upon contentment rather than getting caught up in not having enough or always seeking to have what we perceive others to have. This applies to life and certainly within your pursuit of making teaching yoga feasible and sustainable.

## LOOK UP, NOT OUT

Self-improvement occurs when an upward comparison inspires us to try harder, stay committed, and trust in the process. When it comes to developing as a yoga teacher — and in other aspects of life — I often visualize being on a staircase. The staircase represents the progression we are making through life experiences. As we seek to take that next step up within our growth and development, we keep an eye looking upward toward that next step, extending our hand out to that person who is a little ahead of us so that, with their support, we arrive at the next step along the staircase. At the same time, we are also willing to keep an eye and a hand extended out to support the one who is reaching up to us for support in getting to the step we are on. As yoga teachers, it would be my desire that we would be willing and seek opportunities to come alongside of another teacher and support them in their pursuit of taking the next step. Collectively, we join together. We collaborate, even, to make sure that each of us reaches the next step.

This is a beautiful image that continues to shape my pursuits as a teacher. This approach has allowed me to expand into a growth mindset and approach that supports valuable connection with other teachers and mentors who are aligned within the same intention. This approach doesn't make room for competition or comparison by looking outward instead of upward.

When we look outward, we become distracted and begin to lose sight of our unique purpose and gifts as a teacher. Unhealthy comparison stifles your growth, and you will find yourself stuck and unsure what step you should take next. This outward approach leads to burnout from the hustle of trying to take on too many lateral steps based upon what others are doing. Keeping your focus upward while remaining supportive of others making their way upward at the same time keeps us all moving forward along the staircase rather than clogging up the staircase by remaining stuck on one step.

## UNDERSTAND WHERE YOU ARE

As you make your way toward where you desire to be in your teaching path, it's also important to always acknowledge where you are and what you currently know. Just because another teacher is highly visible on social media with thousands of followers doesn't mean you should necessarily aspire to use that teacher to measure your evolution against. This could actually backfire and push you into imposter syndrome. Look around you and notice those who are a little ahead of you on the teaching pathway and on the next step of the staircase. I would also challenge you to take action to reach out and build a relationship with those people. Instead of judging their growth and experience by what you think you know of them from social posting, reach out and connect to see if you can learn and grow by having a genuine relationship with them. This is one of the reasons I love the mentorship relationship that I have with other teachers so much. Through the mentoring relationship, connections are made, and not only am I able to support other teachers in their teaching experiences, but I am given the opportunity to grow and expand my skill set as a teacher and build interpersonal relationships with others. Through the mentoring relationship, we mutually bring value to each other's experiences and pursuits in the bigger quest of being a yoga teacher. This also affirms to me that we are a collective, and we are in this together, seeking to make a bigger impact on the communities we are serving.

## COMPARE YOURSELF TO YOURSELF

If we begin to view comparison through the lens of using it as a healthy self-evaluation tool, we can then use our experiences to support and formulate lessons, learning what we can take away to get closer to fulfilling our pursuits. I often tell myself and share with other teachers that you will never lead a perfect class. You will have times when you feel inadequate or unsatisfied with your teaching skill set and how you delivered the class experience. You will not always say exactly what you wanted to say or provide the perfect cue. Your transitions will be clunky, and your delivery will fall flat, yet... you can tell yourself, "Next time." This is a powerful self-comparison tool. When those teaching situations occur, because they will, don't revert to self-criticism or judgment—that is unhealthy and doesn't serve you. Instead, make a mental marker and tell yourself, "Next time." Give yourself opportunity within that next class you teach to make an adjustment and to choose to use your past teaching experience as a healthy self-comparison tool.

## DEVELOP SOCIAL MEDIA SAVVY

Begin with building a network of support. Seek connection with others versus comparison. Are you actively making healthy connections, or do you find yourself passively scrolling social media in an attempt to gain clicks and likes that could provide a false sense of connection? Is your time on social media supporting growth and genuine connection, or could your ego be pulling you away from focusing on service as a teacher? Let your time on social media have a direct purpose of building a network of connection.

Consider using your time on social media to seek out and develop relationships like you would offline. Approach social media with an active intention to add value and nourish the community you already have. Get involved and engaged with others who align with your intention for the bigger picture that supports the unique work you are pursuing in service by teaching yoga.

Start conversations and leave only comments of value with a deep desire to expand and grow connection and possibly collaboration. Humans are social in nature, and we are not meant to just scroll through life. We are designed for interaction. Use social media and offline networking opportunities to interact with other teachers and professionals within the community in order to motivate, uplift, and encourage each other within the scope of work and influence you are pursuing teaching yoga.

## PURSUE UPWARD JOY

Joy is a state of being rather than an emotion, such as being happy. Comparison is a fundamental human condition. Instead of generating envy, which is a form of hostility, explore what you admire and appreciate in another individual. Turn unhealthy emotions of comparison and competition into abundance of joy beyond circumstance and a catalyst for personal growth. Reverse the thoughts you have that are directed outward toward someone else and redirect them to inspire and challenge you personally to reflect and inquire into developing and choosing your unique growth strategy and plan of development. Lastly, challenge yourself to see where you are and within your experiences and gifts as a teacher through the lens of joy. The view through this lens will open you up to expand and grow as a teacher in ways that the lens of comparison and completion distorts and obstructs.

## Reflective Exercise

Using the six focal points for avoiding the comparison trap, take a few moments to journal your thoughts on how you will begin to implement each point into your overall growth strategy as an individual and as a yoga teacher.

# Developing Genuine Confidence

---

*"Believe in yourself! Have faith in your abilities! Without a humble but reasonable confidence in your own powers you cannot be successful or happy."*

**— NORMAN VINCENT PEALE**

There is a difference between genuine confidence and superficial confidence. In this lesson, you will learn key signs for distinguishing superficial confidence and how to develop genuine confidence as a yoga teacher.

Why is confidence even important? Well, confidence is attractive. People who exude genuine confidence appeal to and inspire others. Confidence gives people an advantage in all aspects of life, including personal relationships, because confidence is contagious. Interestingly, when someone is confident in their own abilities, others respond by putting confidence in them too. Because of all of these reasons, it is important for yoga teachers to develop genuine confidence. Interestingly, lack of confidence is at the top of the list of obstacles for most yoga teachers I mentor. The great thing is that genuine confidence can be developed.

As we dig deeper into confidence, it will be important to understand that there is a fine line between genuine confidence and pseudo-confidence. When someone crosses that line, their behavior becomes unattractive, which comes across as untrustworthy and phony. Rather than appealing to others, the pseudo-confident person repels others. This persona will most definitely not create connection and will impede your service and impact as a yoga teacher.

## Authentic Vulnerability

Authentic vulnerability is a piece of the development of genuine confidence. Oftentimes when seeking to better understand what something is, it's important, or of great value, to understand what it isn't. To begin understanding genuine confidence and authentic vulnerability, consider the opposite, which is superficial confidence. I'll begin by giving you some characteristics of how superficial confidence might be revealed; from that understanding, you can begin to know better how to develop genuine confidence. Superficial confidence will look like an act or a performance by someone in costume.

Your role is not to step into the yoga classes you lead to deliver a performance reciting a set of rote cues, like the lines of a script. This superficial quality impacts how you speak. You may have even heard the concept of "finding your voice" as a yoga teacher or studied this within your YTT experience. Being a yoga teacher isn't about putting on another persona. It's about being authentically vulnerable, as you are as a person, as well as when you lead yoga practice. Being a yoga teacher should be the natural extension of who you are as a person. Students should encounter you as the teacher in the same way they would encounter you outside the yoga classroom.

Yoga teachers are not in any way to be elevated onto a pedestal or perceived in a guru status. Yoga teachers may be a little farther along in their own experience of the practice, and they may have spent more hours studying or reading yogic texts, but this in no ways denotes superiority. Now, I certainly have great respect for many teachers and the mentors I've had in my life, but I still know that at the end of the day, they are human. It's unfair to put that level of pressure on someone, and it is my hope that, as teachers, we are not fueled by the ego's desire for gratification or status.

## The Myth of Fake It Until You Make It

Let's explore a little more about recognizing superficial confidence through the lens of acting versus being confident. There is a difference, and this is where the statement "fake it until you make it" becomes a big myth. Interestingly, those who act confident struggle to recognize the difference between acting and being confident. But others can easily recognize it.

People with this pseudo-confidence generally dismiss others' reactions to them with statements like "I don't care what people think" or "They're just jealous." This bold projection perpetuates the problem and actually distances others even more. I don't believe this is what anyone truly desires when seeking to develop genuine confidence. It may appear bold, yet it's brash and distancing, maybe even repellant rather than attractive. This appearance is misleading, and once again, it's representative of a putting on an external costume rather than the appearance of genuine confidence that exudes from the inside out.

## Confidence Doesn't Mean You Know Everything

This is a good one. I think right behind a feeling of lack of confidence comes the myth that you must be an expert and know everything in order to be confident. How unrealistic, yet realistic, in the aspect of how we encounter or interact with this concept of being confident. Confidence is based upon a realistic, secure belief in yourself. When you have genuine confidence, you have enough belief in yourself that you are willing to ask questions and seek out and ask for help. A few key words to take note of here are "willing" and "admit." There is an acknowledgment, and this attributes to authentic vulnerability, as well. When it comes to this sense of being confident and being okay with not knowing everything, then you are willing to admit and commit to try and try again until you learn. On the other hand, superficial confidence isn't willing to ask for help or acknowledge the gaps in skill or knowledge. Sadly, superficial confidence is not open or willing to learning or refinement, which will stunt your growth and stifle your development.

## Confidence Doesn't Mean Perfection

Going hand in hand with the acknowledgment of not knowing it all is that confident individuals are not perfect. Confident people make mistakes, accept responsibility, make corrections, learn, and move forward from the mistake. I like to consider mistakes opportunities to learn and grow. Superficial confidence will reveal itself in blaming others rather than accepting responsibility. This mindset will most likely make the same mistakes — or even magnify the mistake — because of an unwillingness to learn, refine, and adjust to move forward. The superficial confident mindset is masked behind "fake it until you make it." This mindset will keep you stuck.

## Confidence Reflects Humility

An individual who embodies genuine confidence doesn't put on airs and finds no need to draw attention to themself. Confident humility relies on substance rather than style. This speaks to the decisions you'll make as to what type of teacher you will be. Superficial confidence seeks attention and will represent itself in an over-the-top or "look at me" approach. Interestingly, the attitude of cockiness and arrogance is simply a mask worn to cover up surface-level confidence. Superficial confidence is threatened by substance. When challenged by difference, superficial confidence is revealed within the actions and attitudes of deflection and defensiveness. Without the depth of substance, a superficial confidence will not hold up to any challenge or scrutiny.

## Confidence is Consistent

Confidence is rooted in consistency that isn't based upon opinion or circumstances. Genuine confidence is unwavering, steady, and ever present. If you feel as though you lack confidence as a teacher, it is important that you are equipped with understanding how to develop genuine confidence. Someone who is confident is not reliant on what others think. Instead, they are content to form their own opinions and to act on their own accord. This type of confidence comes from knowing who you are and what you stand for, anchored in your own values and formed beliefs. Those who are merely acting confident lack the foundation to be consistent and independent because their confidence isn't rooted in values and beliefs. The pseudo-confident individual looks outward for validation and direction. That makes their confidence situational and puts them on shaky ground. That's huge.

As this applies to teaching yoga, if you desire to develop genuine confidence, then you will need to evaluate and seek deeper understanding of what you are trying to teach others. There will come a time when what you were taught in teacher training will need to be evaluated and you will take owner-ship in deciding what your interpretation of the content is and how you will express and share the practice. You will use all that you've learned and gained within training, but through application, you will need to begin to take responsibility for your own understanding. When you have experience and know what you are talking about, your confidence is genuine because it comes from a place you actually know rather than just a place where information was transferred to.

## Confidence Gives Freely and Helps Others

Finally, the last quality of genuinely confident people is that they are also giving of themselves. They see no need to be protective and stingy with their time, knowledge, resources, ideas, or support. They believe there is plenty to go around, and they welcome the opportunity to help others. Genuinely confident individuals seek and see the best in others. They overlook pettiness, forgive, and working earnestly to resolve conflicts. Superficial confidence is guarded and builds walls. Superficially confident individuals isolate themselves and are not forthcoming with information. Yoga teacher, this is where you need to be mindful of falling into the comparison and competition trap discussed in Lesson 10.

There is enough yoga to go around, and no one teacher has the "secret sauce" recipe when it comes to teaching. No one teacher can claim ownership of yoga or make claims on what is real yoga and what is not. This attitude is once again a re-flection of superficial confidence.

Yoga teachers do not need to compete, and we certainly don't need to withhold from helping or supporting each other along the way. This approach will only close off connection and is very destructive to your growth and development as a teacher. Here's where substance over style comes back in. When you have a genuine confidence, you are generous and not consumed with self-serving actions. Unfortunately, when someone remains superficially confident, closed off, and unwilling, they set themselves up for self-sabotage. I have seen this play out, and I have sadly experienced the sting of this attitude and action firsthand within the yoga community.

It is of the utmost importance and integrity that we are in constant acknowledgement of where we are in our development as yoga teachers and that we understand when our confidence becomes skewed and the ego surfaces to boast the superficial qualities of confidence. Guard and equip yourself so that you can remain a solid vessel capable of pouring into and passing along the powerful teachings of yoga to others.

Lastly, at the root of all these behaviors is the difference between genuine confidence and a lack of confidence. Masking a lack of confidence doesn't fool anyone for very long. It soon becomes clear that the pseudo-confident are trying to hide something—usually, a lack of confidence. Just admitting the confidence gap and being confident enough to ask for help resolves this perception and moves people along on the right track toward developing a deeper level of confidence. For some, though, this admission never comes. As a result, these individuals miss out on developing and displaying the genuine confidence that would lead to stronger connections with others. When your connection is weakened, your service as a yoga teacher is impacted, as well.

## Reflective Exercise

Journal your thoughts on the definition of confidence. Using the key points in this lesson for developing genuine confidence, evaluate your definition and whether or not you view confidence differently than it is presented here. What ways can you begin developing genuine confidence today?

# Language that Leads

"If you talk to a man in a language he understands,
that goes to his head. If you talk to him in his
language, that goes to his heart."

— NELSON MANDELA

What you say matters, and how you instruct and lead yoga classes will impact students' experiences in your class. Learn how your verbal and body language, vocal tonality, and the selection of the words you use in class can lead and equip students in creating an autonomous yoga practice. When yoga teachers express to me obstacles they encounter, cueing and sequencing come up often. Both of these are usually at the top of the list, along with a lack of confidence. Now, let's spend some time in this lesson exploring cues and the language used to direct and lead yoga classes.

Why does cueing become an obstacle? Could it be that you find yourself more focused on the sequencing aspect, rather than developing a deeper understanding of how effective cueing and the language you use to lead classes actually become the framework upon which all other aspects of your teaching is built upon?

Just like there is nothing random when it comes to sequencing, the same applies with knowing what to say and when to say it when you teach a yoga class. If you're focused solely on creating sequences without spending time strengthening your language and cues to support a solid foundation, then you'll most likely find yourself questioning whether you're truly leading impactful and meaningful class experiences. You will find yourself hurdling this obstacle over and over again until you lock into the key essentials found within cueing and using language that leads students through a highly effective and successful class experience.

In this lesson, we will explore three key essentials that will support your development in this area of your teaching skill set.

## Effective Communication

Have you ever considered that a huge piece of the technical aspect of being a yoga teacher revolves around how effectively you can communicate. And developing an understanding of what effective communication consists of will fast-track and improve your ability to lead impactful class experiences that are empowering for students.

I want to highlight a few considerations that will support your ability to expand, refine, and grow in this area of your development. This will benefit you greatly not only as a yoga teacher, but also within all communication and relational aspects of your life.

Let's begin with speaking naturally and clearly. I've already expressed the importance of authenticity and how to avoid falling into the trap of imposter syndrome. Part of "finding your voice" as a yoga teacher is not to mimic or replicate someone else but rather to, once again, be yourself. Part of speaking clearly also includes simplicity and limiting the amount of filler words you use. Oftentimes, we aren't even aware of the subconscious words we are using to fill the space. We live in such a stimulus-driven society that there are rarely moments, unless intentionally created, where there isn't some sort of noise or activity filling the spaces we are residing within on a daily basis. Stillness is not a foreign concept within the practice of yoga. Yet, even within the stillness, there is often a juxtaposition of movement present at the same time. What about silence? Rarely do I find spaces where yoga is being taught where there is room for silence. And in our efforts to make practicing yoga appealing and for students to feel inclined to come back to our classes again, teachers and studios feel they should turn the class practice into a production. It often becomes evident that the teacher is consumed with perfecting their class playlist and that they are able to speak all of the narrative they have prepared that the yoga class instruction quickly takes on the dimension of a monologue within a play.

What would happen if we stripped all of that away? Teachers can tune in to the silence and hold that space for students to observe and explore. What would happen if we avoided the need to fill every moment of the class with words, music, and the extra nuances of the experience in an effort to entertain? What if we shifted our teaching focus more toward "how" to practice rather than solely providing an experience?

Without going off course too much with the topic of this lesson, it offers the inquiry of what exactly we are teaching when the teacher's focus relies more heavily on the extras of the experience. Could we be teaching students that these exterior factors are of greater importance than guiding and supporting them to find solace within the interior of their experience?

When you consider avoiding filler words, pay attention to your level of comfort with stillness and silence. It's important that we are not asking students to go somewhere we are not actually exploring and practicing ourselves. This contributes toward diminishing trust between the teacher and student.

I believe that filler words show up for a couple of reasons, which could include the teacher's uncertainty and the teacher being uncomfortable themselves with silence and not fully understanding how to hold that space for the students. It is certainly a process, but once you become more comfortable with releasing any desire or need to talk and consume the space with words, you will begin to create and support the space for the necessary silence that contributes significantly to leading and teaching others how to explore and to become more comfortable within themselves.

Lastly, you'll want to add the layer of tonality within your teaching skill set. What you're saying is of great importance, but the tone you use will have an impact, as well. The tone that you use to deliver the cues and to emphasize your language has the power to invite and support engagement within the experience. Consider this—your cues and language set the framework for the rest of the elements of the class. Although sequencing is definitely a contributing factor in the success of the class experience, it is the cues and language that you use that sets the foundation and provides the framework for the sequences to be placed within.

## Teach Yoga Poses the Same Way—Every Time

There is great beauty within the simplicity of cueing and sequencing. Simplify the cueing process by establishing the framework of understanding that the yoga postures never really end. There is a familiarity, continuity, and thread of corresponding action and expression to be found within every pose. This common thread is found within the acknowledgment and understanding of function, action, and energetic alignment.

Knowing these qualities in Tadasana, Mountain Pose, is essential. When you have a clear understanding of all that is comprised within Mountain Pose, then you can begin to use these attributes as a diagnostic tool for evaluating and accessing every other pose. In essence, Mountain Pose becomes the centerpiece of the yoga asana practice. Teaching students this foundational pose will help to support students in building a sustainable practice and help them connect the dots as they explore and discover the various poses that emerge within the yoga practice sequences you offer.

## Pose Assessment Plan

The concept of reading the pose the same way every time is a piece of your assessment plan. From there, you can begin layering your cues upon that foundation. If your language is not clear and direct—or it becomes hard for you to say—then it will be hard for students to hear, receive, and implement what you are guiding them to experience.

Within your pose assessment plan, you develop and use organizational language and cues that support the creation of form or the shape of the various yoga poses. Form language and cues are comprised of action, muscular engagement and are alignment focused in nature. Once the form begins to emerge, you will blend the use of language that becomes more expressive and organic with qualities of noticing the more subtle aspects of the practice experience. Your pose assessment plan requires you to discern and evaluate the needs of the students you are teaching in real time.

You may find it is more beneficial to rely more heavily on the language of organization and form until you sense that the connection is being made within the learning experience of the practice. You then begin to explore offering language and directives that invite inquiry and qualities of curiosity for the students to explore as they begin to evaluate how they are being, in addition to what they are doing, as they create and experience the various yoga pose shapes. Ultimately, as you begin to use your pose assessment plan on a consistent basis, you will become better equipped to discern and offer the appropriate guidance to support the practice experience you are leading.

## Bridge the Gap

Within the framework of cueing, all other aspects of the class are built. Oftentimes, teachers rely more heavily of the creative aspect of sequencing when the priority of preparation begins with the solid framework of the cues and language used to lead the class. This framework not only supports a strong foundation upon which the class is built but also bridges the gap for students between the external and internal experience. Keep it simple. Consider gleaning your language and providing three clear and direct cues per pose and on each side. Seek to use language and provide cues that are easy to understand and follow.

## Reflective Exercise

Record audio of yourself teaching and take your own class. Notice the cues and directives you are using. Are your words and directives clear and understandable? Reflect and journal upon what students might actually be hearing with the language you use to lead classes, rather than solely what you desire to say.

# Leading Students to Discover Autonomy

---

"The art of teaching is the art of assisting discovery."
— MARK VAN DOREN

In this lesson, we'll explore what autonomy is and how the teacher's focus and intention has a direct impact upon offering an autonomous experience for students. As a teacher, you will either equip and empower others to trust their own intuitive agency and guidance, or you will teach students to attach to the surface aspects of the practice that makes them dependent on you for continual guidance. Learn key words for inviting autonomy in class.

## Autonomy Defined

Autonomy is the idea of self-direction, and it's generally understood as referring to the capacity to be one's own person. It is the concept of living one's life according to one's own reasons and motives, not according to external forces that could be dictated, manipulated, or distorted. Autonomy includes independence, responsibility, and ownership. There's an idea that we are all born with an inner driving force.

To understand that part of our role is to guide and lead others to develop and experience their own unique experience within the yoga practice setting, we must question the constructs or organization of the traditional yoga class setting we are most accustomed to, especially in the Western approach to teaching yoga in a studio setting. This traditional setting has become commonplace, but is it distorting the potential impact that the teachings of yoga can have on the students? Many YTTs focus on individuals memorizing then repeating a set script or class sequence without placing much emphasis or thoughts toward why the sequence was arranged the way it was.

I have had many conversations with teachers who have completed a YTT program, only to find they really weren't confident in the sequencing approach they were taught—and this makes stepping out of the training to lead others very challenging. This rote memorization approach does not equip new teachers with a strong understanding of the foundational structure of sequencing and the language that supports the delivery of this experience.

## Sequence for Success

Without a clear foundational understanding for organizing and leading a class experience that includes a solid structure, as well as the in-depth analysis of spontaneity that comes when teaching real-time class experiences, many trainees and new yoga teachers can quickly become overwhelmed when the ideal student they prepared their sequence for doesn't show up. This is why it is very important that YTT programs equip trainees with the understanding of adapting and adjusting their sequence structure so that they can meet the needs of the actual students who attend their class.

The concept of autonomy support, as given by a yoga teacher, accounts for the psychological needs of the students and the collective class, extending well beyond the appearance or shape of the yoga poses. Rather than the practice experience being a dictation or dissertation given by the teacher, the class setting can become more like a dialogue that includes meaningful feedback, choices, and encouragement given by the teacher. Consider the class experience as one that sets students up for success in the development of listening closer to their unique needs. Moments of celebration support the realization of the students' inner capacity to choose and create the experience they wish to have on their yoga mat. That translates out to the creation of the life they wish to live. Autonomy supports this success.

## Understanding Motivation

Tucked within the ability for yoga teachers to lead others toward the creation of an autonomous experience is the understanding of what drives us to step back onto the yoga mat. Motivation gives us many valuable insights into human nature. It explains why we set goals, strive for achievement, and desire psychological intimacy and connection. This is also why we experience emotions like fear, anger, and compassion. Motivation helps us understand how to relate to our emotions and develop this sense of returning back to joy and nurturing the relational aspect of our being. All of this shows up within the yoga practice.

Learning about motivation is valuable because it supports our understanding of where it comes from, why it changes, and what causes it to increase and decrease while also providing the understanding for how to adapt to the aspects that cannot be controlled or changed. Ultimately, this deeper understanding helps us answer the question of why some types of motivation are more beneficial than others.

Motivation contributes toward autonomy in that it reflects something unique about each of us and offers valuable insight into our personal growth. It becomes a pathway to shift and alter our way of thinking, feeling, and behaving. Motivation aligns with our mindset. For the yoga teacher, this aspect of understanding equips you in the development of the relational aspect of teaching that you will need as you seek to meet students where they are, to support their needs, and ultimately to support the autonomous practice experience that will draw students back.

## Choose Your Words Wisely

There is an element of uncertainty when beginning to teach from a place that provides choice and responsibility. It will serve you well to establish and reinforce a strong foundational structure for sequencing and leading classes. You need a class plan. You also need to develop spontaneity. You must choose to empty yourself of the need to cling to the rigidity of the plan so that you can see the people you are leading. Pay close attention and be cautious within the space you hold as you lead a yoga practice. Understand the space you're holding and the impact that the space fosters has on the students who practice there. Consider your language and choose your words wisely. Place emphasis on leading with language that encourages students to create a fresh encounter in the practice as they listen to the intuitive intelligence and guidance within them. Prompt them to notice. Words and phrases that invite and prompt curiosity—such as notice, consider, or I invite you—will support a class environment that allows students to choose for themselves what they sense and need with the practice experiences.

## Reflective Exercise

Journal the cues you use in class. Write out the action that your words and directives are inviting. Evaluate whether your language is leading and promoting autonomy for students or projecting a perceived experience you desire students to have.

Evaluate what motivates you to teach. When you step out of yoga teacher training, you have a big decision to make, and you will evaluate and re-evaluate it often. What type of teacher are you going to be? What type of teacher are you going to commit to developing into?

# The Importance of Feedback

---

"Knowledge rests not upon truth alone, but upon
error also."

– CARL JUNG

In this lesson, the concept of feedback is defined. The lesson
will also discuss the importance of timing, how to offer feedback, what to suggest as feedback, whom you should ask for
feedback from, and the willingness to receive, process, and
apply feedback.

There is a great relational aspect to teaching. Besides the
teacher-student relationship, teachers develop relationships
with their fellow teachers, studio and gym owners, and various others. Teachers must also consider how they relate to the
practice of yoga.

As a yoga teacher, you will find yourself immersed in these
interactions. Interestingly, through various conversations I
have had with other teachers, I have found that yoga teachers
can also feel lonely at times and uncertain whom they can turn
to or call upon for guidance. I highly encourage you to seek
out a mentor and to establish this relationship, as it will have
a great impact on your success and longevity as a teacher.

As you begin to teach and evaluate your teaching experiences for the purpose of refinement, it is my hope that this
lesson will support you in connecting the dots between the
feedback tool and the impact this has on your relationships,
as well. Feedback and refinement become powerful tools not

only in relating to others but in becoming more aware and in-tune with your relationship to yourself, as an individual, and as a yoga teacher.

I'll begin by sharing about a teaching experience I had early in my teaching career. I had been teaching for maybe two years at this time, and I was presented with the opportunity to teach at a new yoga studio in the area. This would be my first teaching position outside of a gym or YMCA setting. I was a bit nervous yet very excited about the opportunity to grow as a teacher in a new setting. I was also grateful for the opportunity given to me by the studio owner, who would eventually become a lifelong friend and mentor to me. Her name is Wanda. The development of this relationship has impacted my life in a variety of ways beyond my role as a yoga teacher. Her leadership and guidance supported me then, and our relationship continues to thrive as we have shared many life experiences over the years as teachers, mothers, and friends. I have no doubt that her guidance and influence, especially during that season that I shared supporting the studio she owned, has impacted my ability to develop and grow, finding my own unique path of service and passion as a teacher for over two decades now.

I'm not exactly sure when it occurred, but one day, I came in to teach my scheduled class and who did I find in my class? Wanda. Needless to say, my heart began to beat a little faster, and I became nervous. Honestly, her presence was a bit intimidating. I had such respect for her, and it was an honor to have her as a student in my class. I quickly organized myself and led the class. Now, here is the part I want you to pay close attention to, as this is the focus this lesson revolves around. After the class, Wanda graciously provided me feedback. Her feedback was constructive, yet filled with love and full of her highest intent to support me and to see me succeed stepping into my power and fullness as a yoga teacher.

## The Importance of Feedback

If you are a studio owner, or desire to eventually be one, then I highly encourage you to equip and train your teaching and support staff with this powerful tool of refinement. This will not only create cohesion and comradery among your staff but ultimately support the bigger picture—supporting the communities you serve by providing the highest value of an experience found within the setting of a yoga class. Feedback helps to support clear expectations. If you lead a yoga teacher training program, I would highly suggest that you equip trainees with this impactful tool so that they can place it in their yoga teacher toolbox and carry it with them as they venture out pursuing their personal development and growth strategy as a teacher.

In order to find relevance and value in feedback, it is also important to understand the meaning behind the use of this tool and how to apply it. Constructive feedback should also provide the opportunity to support another individual from a positive intention to identify growth opportunities that they might not see as easily in themselves.

## The Balance of Giving and Receiving

Feedback has both a giving and a receiving aspect. For the tool of feedback to function as designed, one must understand the responsibility involved within giving constructive feedback, as well as receiving feedback constructively. The word constructive is defined as "serving a useful purpose; tending to build up." Finding clarity in this word's meaning will guide the giver toward constructive feedback, but it will also impact the recipient of feedback. When both parties understand the responsibility involved with feedback, this supports the value and impact of the feedback.

## Timing is Everything

Let's dig into some key points for giving constructive feedback, along with points on how to prepare to receive and apply feedback. I have found that when I am going to give another teacher feedback that timing is everything. When it comes to leading a yoga class and holding space energetically for the learning experience that takes place in that setting, it is important to give space for the teacher to absorb the teaching experience afterward and finish tending to the needs of the students and responsibilities that come with wrapping up the class in the teaching space. Just like other situations in life, the time in which we initiate an action or a response will have a big impact on the effectiveness of the delivery and how well it is received.

I have found that when ample time is given to first process the teaching experience, from the perspective of what the student has experienced, and then from the perspective of teaching, then I am able to collect, organize and thoughtfully gather clear, direct, and beneficial points of refinement that will support the teacher I'm offering feedback to. I choose to acknowledge the gift and guidance of the practice experience. I prefer to give feedback in a written format so that my words can be chosen thoughtfully, edited, and shared more wisely. When I give feedback from this approach, I feel like I have truly given the individual the very best intentional support I can offer. For me, giving space between the class and the feedback is appropriate. This will also give the teacher time to prepare to receive the feedback and process in their own timing, which most likely is not right after a class or while they are trying to wrap up and take care of their responsibilities that conclude when they are making their way to the parking lot to leave.

What if you are asked to provide feedback? Do you have a method or process in place that prepares you to give constructive feedback? Do you know how to give feedback in a way that will be effective and beneficial for the one who is asking?

There is a level of discernment involved when you find yourself in a situation where feedback would greatly benefit the teacher, yet you're not quite sure how they will receive your feedback. In this case, you must evaluate and discern whether or not the timing is right and whether or not this individual is ready to receive feedback. If you're not sure, then one way to find out is to simply ask if they are open to receiving your feedback. If they are, give it intentionally.

In some cases, you may discern that your feedback would benefit a teacher you have not yet developed a relationship with. In this case, offering feedback might not be beneficial, especially if you are not in a position to follow up with this individual after giving feedback.

## Asking for Feedback

How do you ask for feedback? In some studios or spaces where you will teach, the concept of feedback may already be a part of the teaching staff's process. Studio leadership may have various methods and processes in place for how they initiate, receive, and implement feedback. When you agree to take on a teaching position, it is important that you understand this expectation or ask if this is a part of the ongoing development of the teaching staff. If a feedback system is not in place or is not offered regularly, then I encourage you to independently seek out and ask for feedback on your own so that you might begin implementing this impactful tool into your ongoing growth strategy.

## What to Offer and How to Offer Feedback

The concept of feedback can feel or become vast because there could be many things to offer or say about the practice experience, and if not thoughtfully considered, the information shared could become subject to personal preference. Just as there is a vastness to the cues and informational directives we offer to students within the class practice setting, a best practice would be to use restraint when acknowledging or offering feedback. If your intent is to provide positive support, acknowledgement, and guidance, then choose your words wisely and limit them so that the key points of feedback can actually be heard and received well.

A few key points that would serve another teacher well would include:

- The pacing, rhythm, or tempo of the class.
- Tone and volume of the teacher's voice.
- Use of clear and direct language and cues of instruction.
- The presence of the teacher, including the felt sense of being seen as a student, and that needs were supported and met.

I would steer clear of feedback that is preference-oriented or pertains to the teacher's style. Keeping the feedback oriented toward the technical aspect will be more beneficial than offering aesthetic-oriented points. I have found that suggestions that can be applied to the next class are more beneficial than feedback referring to an isolated experience where the teacher might not be able to alter the situation or offer the class experience differently.

How do you offer feedback? I always start by acknowledging the gift of the experience and acknowledging understanding of the courage it takes to put oneself in the role of teacher, in the spotlight of delivering and holding the space for the practice experience. I then offer points that a teacher should consider continuing to implement and provide in the practice. I include points that made the experience unique and special according to the skill sets that I felt the particular teacher really excelled within. I then offer specific points that will support the teacher's ability to implement and explore within the next class they teach. Be specific with this feedback. These points might include the overuse of filler words or unclear cues or possibly cues of alignment and actions that could create safety concerns if they continue to be offered. Other important points of feedback would be how the space felt to me as a student, whether the environment invited exploration in the practice experience, and whether time was properly allocated to savasana.

These points, to me, are nonnegotiable. These points aren't about preference. They support the fullness of the experience beyond preference. They are requirements for all yoga teachers to support and hold with the highest integrity of the yoga practice experience.

## Willingness to Receive

Let's explore an important aspect of feedback—how to prepare to receive feedback. This is important, and it begins with being willing to receive feedback. It is key for you to be able to absorb and apply what you are being given. If you understand you are being given constructive feedback that is supportive and positive, then it becomes a valuable gift of refinement. A big part of cultivating a willing heart and attitude toward receiving feedback comes from giving yourself an ego check regularly. You are not going to be open to receiving feedback if your ego is in the way. Your ego will be a barrier to receiving and growing. Your ego will tell you that you don't need feedback.

So check your ego. You don't know everything. You aren't going to know everything, and if you truly desire to create longevity and sustainability within growth as an individual and as a yoga teacher, then you will also want to work on clearing that space within yourself so that you can be open to an expanded version of yourself. This will require refinement, and for that, you will need feedback from trusted teachers and mentors. If you are not open to feedback, then you will actually constrict your ability to grow in your teaching skill set. When you're open to feedback, you will move beyond the limited view that your ego will want you to believe and experience.

## Feedback Plan

As I wrap up this lesson, I want to share with you a tangible way to implement a feedback system. A dear friend, and fellow teacher shared this plan with me and it has proven to be quite beneficial when implemented. If you are a studio owner, this would be a great system of support to implement within the development of your teaching staff. This plan will also support you with some self-feedback when you are feeling uninspired or wondering why your classes have low attendance. The following feedback action plan will support you with some key points to evaluate. I encourage you to use this plan consistently to keep yourself aligned with your desired growth strategy as a teacher. This plan also supports the relationship you have with the leadership and ownership of the spaces in which you teach, such as the studio owners and group fitness managers. This is an action that communicates you care about your personal growth, and it speaks volumes that you are willing to learn, or unlearn in some cases, so that you can contribute greater toward upleveling the class experience you are offering for the students you support and serve.

Here's the plan. Think of it as a growth action plan. Use the acronym FAST. It can be broken down as follows:

## F – Follow Up

Ask yourself, "Have I followed up with the new students in my class and the students who attend my class regularly? Who have I not seen in a while?" Take action to reach out in whatever way seems authentic to you and in accordance with communicating to students within the spaces you teach.

## A – Ask and Apply

Have I asked for and/or applied feedback from other teachers and teaching mentors? Use discernment in choosing who you ask, as well. Not everyone has developed the understanding of how to effectively offer and receive feedback.

## S – Simplify

Have I made my sequencing or class structure too complicated? Am I sequencing and leading with simplicity within my sequence and the cues I'm offering?

## T – Take

Have I taken other teachers' classes? Am I taking workshops or additional trainings to support my growth as a teacher?

Understanding how to give and receive constructive feedback isn't complicated. Work to cultivate an attitude and heart that is ready to receive feedback. Certainly, as with all situations in life, there may be times when the feedback does not come from a constructive and positive place. It happens. In those instances, I would suggest thanking the individual for offering while releasing any need to defend yourself. You can receive the feedback graciously with gratitude and nothing more. You can then choose whether or not you will process and apply that feedback. Remember, constructive feedback is a great refinement tool. Approach and give feedback with an attitude of support and a willingness to receive.

## Reflective Exercise

Evaluate your perspective on feedback and what that process currently means to you within your development and growth as a yoga teacher. Consider seeking out a mentor who can support you by providing valuable feedback and accountability loop within your development as a yoga teacher. Begin to develop and implement FAST within your growth strategy.

# Becoming an Agent of Change

---

"Seek to make peace with change."

— SANDY RAPER

To be an effective yoga teacher is to be an agent of change. This lesson will define the mechanics of change and discuss how a yoga teacher can support students in using the yoga practice to understand areas of resistance and how to cultivate effective and appropriate responses on and off the mat in order to make necessary life changes and ultimately make peace with the changes that occur in life.

The Yoga Sutras of Patanjali begins with the phrase, "Now, the practice of yoga." The word now indicates a consequence and is used to draw the reader's attention to emphasize what is to come. It's as if he's telling us, "Wait for it."

I also find it interesting that even in this ancient text this call to action was necessary. Such is the plight of humanity. First of all, there is a need to recognize the human condition of mental suffering from the habits of our minds. From this recognition, Patanjali then begins to lay out the path of yoga that provides a system that moves us toward realization and the ultimate release and elimination of suffering that we, as humans, are really good at heaping upon ourselves.

If we are to understand more fully our condition — our "problem," you can call it — then the path, or solution, we pursue will be viewed from the lens of remembering our capacity to make appropriate responses to life circumstances and situations that begins to lessen the suffering that comes through reactive thought and action. Through the ongoing pursuit and spiritual quest to seek appropriate responses to the choices we make daily, and within every moment, we begin to acknowledge and implement the practices of yoga into our daily living. We can then begin to lessen the reactive nature that once so easily ensnared us in this habitual trap of suffering.

Let's go back to the word now. "Now what?" you might ask. Patanjali sets out on a mission to lay it all out for us. He gives us a plan and provides structure. The plan of yoga is the realization that in order to remain consistent, without reactive thoughts and actions, amid the ongoing flux of change, then the ongoing pursuit will be required so that we can respond to the habitual patterns of suffering we create when we resist change by seeking permanence in life. Change is the only constant.

This lesson explores how understanding change is part of your role as a yoga teacher. Your role is vital in inviting others to implement Patanjali's Eight-limbed Path into their pursuits of practicing yoga. This is really what you offer to students each and every time you step in to lead a yoga practice. In essence, your role as teacher is to continually remind students of their capacity to respond appropriately — until they remember that for themselves. Ironically, you yourself, as teacher, are in the process of learning and growing within this same system and plan of yoga. The ongoing, daily pursuit to eliminate the habits of suffering are yours to explore at the same time as you lead others in the discovery, as well. What an endeavor and journey to embark upon!

In order to prepare for this endeavor, you must equip yourself with some tools and supplies before you step out onto this journey we often call the yoga practice. If you want to teach and share with students from a place of authentic integrity, you must commit to leading by example. Can we really justify the methodology and pursuit of service teaching yoga if we're asking students to commit to a practice that we aren't actually committing to ourselves? If we aren't practicing what we teach, then it just doesn't line up. Our teaching will not pour out from a place of congruency and integrity, and students will notice.

## Defining Change

If you are resolute in your role as an agent of change teaching yoga then you should first become familiar with what change is, how it happens, and how to share and offer others guidance along the pathway of practicing yoga. This pathway ultimately leads others toward the teacher who resides within them. To walk this pathway is to become supported and well-equipped with guidance from a teacher while using the lessons of life experience and remembering one's own capacity to choose the appropriate response repeatedly. Of course, it is certainly nice to continue to seek guidance from others who are teaching that might share a nugget of wisdom from their experience while not becoming reliant or dependent upon a teacher in order to move forward in your own understanding.

As yoga teachers and yoga practitioners, if we truly believe in the teachings of yoga and the residue of transformation that comes from sustaining the practice, then we will seek to become as effective as we can at sharing with others. In this way, they, too, can equip themselves with the tools and teachings to implement yoga into their daily lives and make peace with change themselves.

So what happens when we encounter change—mentally, physically, and emotionally—in our life through the practice of yoga? Well, if we can begin to understand how to take notice of change, we can also begin to better understand how to sustain it.

## Resistance

Within the concept of change is an element of resistance. Resistance to change is a normal reaction, and we can encounter resistance in a variety of ways. I think sometimes the word resistance can be interpreted in a solely negative aspect when, in fact, resistance is a great communicator and indicator of what is going on within us both physically and mentally. Resistance is also a great evaluation tool and can be used and applied when we find ourselves in the process of change.

### WAKE UP

If resistance is a good communicator, then what exactly is it trying to communicate to us? Well, first, it's trying to get our attention. Resistance is a wake-up call. I can remember early in my practice how physically I began to feel the asana and how it showed up in a variety of ways. The yoga asana practice was unlike any other movement modality I had encountered. It was definitely an attention-getter. And It also piqued my curiosity, because within the sensations and resistance that I felt, there was the layer of awakening that sparked my interest to know more. This drew me back to the next class and the next. Resistance can communicate a pursuit of inquiry, a need or desire to know more. It becomes an invitation to understand better, more fully, how we are moving in our bodies and how we are being in that tricky and pesky space in our minds where the swirling thoughts and stories reside.

Resistance and this invitation to explore also comes with a choice. We can choose to explore, or we can choose to ignore, staying within the default pattern of what feels comfortable and known. We can choose to shut down and not feel. You have probably heard that saying about growth and your comfort zone — our ability to grow and expand becomes dependent on our willingness to step out of our comfort zone. Lastly, we can choose to wake up.

## Communicate Change

How do yoga teachers communicate this aspect and better understanding of change? And how do we communicate and educate others on how to sustain the ever-present constant of change both on their yoga mats and in their lives?

This is more than how to cue the class. When you step into the space of a yoga class to lead students toward and through the experience of yoga, how effectively are you being an agent of change? This goes beyond the technical aspect of teaching and taps into the relational aspect of being a yoga teacher. How prepared are you in your own personal dedication and practice? How grounded are you in knowing and interacting with all eight-limbs of the yoga practice for yourself?

The even bigger question to ponder is, do you wholeheartedly believe that yoga can offer transformation and sustaining change? Immediately, this might seem like a no-brainer question to answer, but I would venture to say that many teachers struggle with confidence (half of the teachers I mentor will attest to this), and part of this lack of confidence is most likely because you're not quite sure if you wholeheartedly believe in the capacity for yoga to offer the transformation. You might not have experienced this transformative change yourself. If that's the case, then sit with this for a few moments, or a season if need be. Lessen doubt in yourself as a teacher and instead choose and use this revelation to cast some light on this area of where you are in your relationship with the yoga practice. Allow this revelation to communicate what you must learn and explore so that you know the practice for yourself more fully. Then use this time of excavation and discovery to communicate and share the practice with more confidence and ease.

## Lasting Change

Stop and think about the title of this section. Is lasting change a paradox, or could it be that bettering our understanding of the process of change can make a lasting impact on our lives and change the trajectory of our paths in life? Choices and change go together. When we figure out how to respond appropriately and repeatedly, we begin to navigate new pathways in our minds. Those comfortable ruts that we had found ourselves in within the habits of our minds, the ones that create suffering, start to lessen, and we begin to find ourselves within the flow of life instead.

Sometimes we get ourselves bogged down thinking that change has to be this big, life-altering experience. Quite honestly, from my own experience, lasting change is more subtle. Although big life changes do occur, it is within the small adjustments and adaptations made within the intuitive interior space of my being that ultimately change my interaction with life.

## Supporting Change

Lastly, when it comes to sustaining change and becoming an agent of change as a yoga teacher, a level of support is needed for change to occur. Sounds easy, huh? You could think of this as a sense of allowing. This is where the aspect of making peace with change begins to emerge. You are allowing a space that is supportive for the condition of change to be nurtured, nourished, and explored without judgment. We begin to notice and then begin to give ourselves permission and support. We also seek others as a layer of relational support. We seek others who are on the same path, and we come to realize that we collectively, as part of humanity, are all in this thing we call life together. There is great comfort to be found in this realization, and hope emerges again to remind us we are capable of cultivating change.

In order to sustain and create lasting change, we must approach it with flexibility and patience. I'm not talking about the physical flexibility that we find in the yoga asana practice but the mental and emotional pliability that supports and equips us to make peace with change. When we can develop this understanding, we are able to cultivate longevity within whatever circumstances present themselves. We will be equipped and ready to adapt. It's not a matter of whether change will happen; it's a question of what you will do when it does.

## Reflective Exercise

Set a timer and have a seat. Spend some time in silent meditation. Observe the fluctuations of your mind and how you respond to the changes that take place within your time of meditation. Journal your meditation experience, reflecting and noticing your reactions and responses. Evaluate how you respond to life changes and situations throughout your day, week, and month. Commit to doing this often.

# Five Keystone Habits for Yoga Teachers

---

"Keystone habits offer what is known within academic literature as 'small wins.' They help other habits to flourish by creating new structures, and they establish cultures where change becomes contagious."

**– CHARLES DUHIGG**

Keystone habits are the small routine actions that we take daily that make a significant impact in all areas of life. In this lesson, learn five keystone habits to incorporate and implement daily that will have a huge impact on the development of confidence, character, and leadership as a yoga teacher.

In this lesson, I want to introduce the concept of keystone habits and how impactful these habits can be within development of becoming a highly effective yoga teacher. These habits will benefit you in any aspect of life. The development of the keystone habits will not only impact you, but also trickle out into the yoga classroom. The dedicated implementation of keystone habits will lead you toward becoming the teacher you desire to be.

When you step out of teacher training, you will know enough to start your teaching journey. Begin to teach what you know, and then from there, you set out to teach what you need to learn further. Although your yoga teacher training is a crucial starting point, it is just the beginning. YTT is definitely a catalyst for discovery and transformation, but the process of becoming is much more detailed—it requires dedication and hard work. This isn't taught during YTT, though. Like other commitments in life, you must evaluate whether you are willing to put in the work, to show up for yourself and others, and ultimately let the teacher within you reveal itself in the timing that is needed. Patience is involved because this aspect of becoming could take a while.

Our society and the lifestyles we've become accustomed to don't really support that mentality, though. When we want something, we get it—almost instantly. And yoga teachers are not immune to this. I believe we translate this mentality into our growth and development as teachers, as well. We become disillusioned and even frustrated because we feel like we should instantaneously become an experienced teacher upon completing YTT. The completion certificate is only an acknowledgement of the beginning of a much longer process.

So, how do keystone habits fit into all of this? They will support you in the process of becoming the teacher you envision and desire to be. As you find yourself farther along in the process, you will most likely add to this list of keystone habits, but I will begin with the following five.

## Community

The development of community in your life will support you greatly and in a variety of ways. When you think about the word community, start small. Think about who you have in your inner circle. This could be one person or up to five individuals. Define who these key people are in your life who will support your work and commitment toward becoming a yoga teacher. Define the people who support you outside of your role of teaching yoga, as well. It's important to access the big picture of life and establish a network and build relationships to immerse yourself within.

For me, my family and my faith community has been a bedrock and continues to support and ground me. From there, the extension of community reaches into the realm of my becoming a yoga teacher. Although these communities have overlap, I have found great relationships of community not in just one particular area. When you think about your community supporting you in your pursuit of teaching, expand outward from that inner circle. Cultivate community within the relationships you have with other teachers, studio and gym owners, and other professionals you encounter as a yoga teacher. The relationships you establish and support with fellow teachers should become another ring around the sphere of your influence that encases your small inner circle of community.

Once you identify your community, invest in these relationships on a daily basis. Seek genuine encounters. Here is where the habit begins to develop and grow. Ask yourself what you can do on a daily or weekly basis to cultivate and nurture these relationships. Commit to holding yourself aligned within this identity group by evaluating how you are showing up in growing these healthy relationships in your community as a yoga teacher. We are hardwired for connection, so it makes sense that we would seek to make it a habit in developing, maintaining, and supporting these connections to thrive in our lives.

It's important to set realistic and attainable habits. It may take some extra effort initially, but soon the byproduct of the keystone habits you establish will trickle into your everyday living. Then they will no longer be a have to but become a must have.

Establishing keystone habits isn't about setting goals. This is different. This is about evaluating the processes and systems you currently have in place and then adjusting and adapting so that you can implement and commit, with consistency, to taking action to apply these habits. Take action daily to nurture and nourish your community in some way. It may be through a personal interaction with your inner circle. It may be an interaction with your broader community. If you have built a social media community or an email newsletter list that follows you and your teaching pursuits, then ask yourself daily and weekly how consistent you have been in nurturing those relationships. How are you showing up for those who follow you?

It becomes more about relationship than numbers at that point. You will begin to attract those who align with you and the community you are building when you implement this approach. And think about this—if you aren't consistently nurturing the audience you currently have, then adding more will not develop the relational aspect of teaching that is vital for your success and longevity as a teacher.

## Spend Time Alone

Solitude isn't a foreign concept for yoga practitioners. Yet as teachers, we can become distracted when we begin teaching and equate the time that we are leading and teaching to our personal practice time. The time that you dedicate to your personal relationship and experiential learning as a student is a powerful space of insight for you as a teacher. This time is for you and should be dedicated solely to your deeper understanding. The commitment you make to this time comes from the intention that is separate from giving or sharing with others. It isn't forced. Instead, it becomes a storehouse where intuitive intelligence resides. When setting out to make time alone and develop this keystone habit, get intentional and even commit to a designated time daily when you will meet with yourself.

In my house, I love to be the first one to get up, because this is time that I capture and spend alone. It's a time I gift to myself, and it's become precious. As the day gets going and others in my house begin to move around with the activities of the day, the space of stillness and solitude feels less accessible. It hasn't always been this way for me. Several years back, I had to become very intentional and create this habit, which required a shift in my schedule. My schedule, or system, I had in place at that time was lacking the structure I needed to make spending time alone accessible. I had also begun to feel like it was taking longer for me to get going in the mornings. Then before I knew it, hours had passed, and it was quickly lunchtime. I could feel and notice that a change was needed. I choose then to commit to getting up at the same time every day. Usually, my day starts at five thirty in the morning. It works for me, and it gives me the time alone and space that I now crave. It has become that must-have to start my day. When that doesn't happen, the day feels somewhat off for me.

As a yoga teacher, I also hear from others that time alone can be foreign to others. Quite honestly, some people find spending time alone uncomfortable and possibly fear what they might encounter during the time when they are alone. It is uncharted territory. And for yoga teachers, it can feel the same way. I'm going to encourage you to commit to what is possible with consistency. As a yoga teacher, you will be inviting others to experience all facets of the practice, including stillness and alone time. Your authenticity is of great importance so that you know, from experience, where you are leading others.

Check your current approach toward stillness or time alone and see if you are giving yourself enough time and space to encounter this daily. If not, make the necessary adjustments to your schedule. I have no doubt that you will find that implementing and developing this keystone habit will have a trickle effect into all areas of your life and, in particular, your pursuit of becoming a yoga teacher.

## Study

Dedicate to studying or learning something new on a daily basis. This doesn't apply solely to yoga. There are many great resources within many aspects of our lives where what we learn can be applied and infused into our role of becoming a yoga teacher. Every book I read, every podcast and sermon I listen to, I am evaluating and processing the implication of what I'm hearing or learning into my daily living. This new learning ultimately makes its way into my role as a yoga teacher. What are you seeking to learn and know more about when it comes to enhancing your skills as a teacher?

Discernment is of great value within the development of the keystone habit of study. Beware of falling into the trap of jumping from one training to the next or piling on knowledge for the sake of knowledge without ever applying what you are learning. Application is integral within this keystone habit of study. Acquiring credentials or training certificates is great as long as they are adding value to the teaching aspect of what you are offering versus consuming more knowledge without a clear plan and direction for utilizing what you have learned. This can be an easy trap to fall into, leading to burnout as you try to convince yourself that you will be ready once you have the next latest and greatest training certificate.

The keystone habit of study is not a quest for acquiring more and more knowledge. I often encourage new teachers to get the practical and real-time experience of teaching first and then spend time evaluating what sparks their interest in studying or learning more. Let that inquiry guide your decisions on what your next course of study or training will entail.

## Application and Integration

The next keystone habit to explore goes hand in hand with the habit of study. Create a habit of integrating what you are learning by actually applying and teaching the new concept or information you've gathered. What really works well for me it to dissect a concept or approach that I am studying and then seek to put the pieces back together into the wholeness of that new aspect of knowledge. This approach has served me well over the years as some of the content of learning that we dive into, as teachers, can become quite vast and dense at the same time. If a strategy of application and integration is not well-thought-out and applied, then you can quickly find yourself submerged in the vastness and possibly become overwhelmed and entangled in the weeds of wondering what to even do with all the knowledge you are consuming. The concept of "teaching what we need to learn" supports the further development of this keystone habit.

If we desire to know anatomy more, then we need to start learning, infusing, and adding the cues and language that support this learning into the class experiences we lead. Experiential learning adds a greater opportunity of applied knowledge becoming wisdom. You don't have to know it all or be an expert to begin teaching small incremental pieces of anatomy, alignment, or whatever concept it may be. Start with one pose and give the instructions and guidance that supports the ability for the student to connect the dots in anatomical reality and enhance or even elevate their experience as they practice yoga.

## Challenge Yourself

The last keystone habit in this lesson is to challenge yourself. Although it is easy to stay in our comfort zone, that can also be stifling. Comfort will stunt your growth. The other keystone habits will be less effective if you aren't willing to devote yourself fully to this one. Certainly there is a place for comfort and ease in our lives. We often hear the balance of effort and ease that supports a fullness of life spoken of within the practice of yoga. Our brains and minds are always going to seek to take the easy path or easy way out. In order to find growth, expansion, or success in anything we do, we must also be willing to be uncomfortable and okay with not knowing clearly how it all plays out.

Trust is involved, along with the understanding of our capacity to be uncomfortable within the growing and learning phases of our lives. I have often trained teachers who want me to tell them exactly what to do and what their teaching path will look like. They want to know that at the end of the training, they will be set up with a full teaching schedule and that teaching yoga will be all they had envisioned it to be. Well, it doesn't happen that way. Life doesn't play out that way, so why would the path of teaching be any different?

Even in my own personal teaching experiences, I never could've fully anticipated some of the amazing teaching opportunities I have been able to take part in. My own expectations would have limited me. I have found that through an openness to explore, to step out of my comfort zone, and to be challenged to teach a variety of classes to a variety of individuals with uniquely different needs from the practice, I have been able to grow and expand. Ultimately, this is how I became the teacher I am today.

When it comes to teaching, I am at ease because of the challenges I have been willing to take. After more than two decades, I still do not know all there is to know about the practice of yoga. I have not arrived, and that is not the goal. I do not dare to think otherwise, because there is still so much more to experience, to learn, and now, to also unlearn. The willingness to say yes to teaching opportunities that weren't within a predictable setting and meeting people where they are within their understanding has gifted me with the ability to cultivate a relational skill set as a teacher. That allows me to make the practice accessible to all who venture into the practice setting. Has it been comfortable? No. Have I fumbled my way through teaching situations? Yes. Have all of my teaching experiences given value to my overall development as a teacher? Most definitely! But I had to choose — to be okay with the uncomfortable and sometimes clunky experiences because I knew that through the discomfort, I would grow and have the opportunity and experiences I did not want to miss out on.

You might find that you already have several of these keystone habits in place. If that's the case, then I want to challenge you to evaluate the systems and processes you currently have in place for each of these. Ask yourself where you might be able to expand and grow within each habit. Notice where you have become comfortable and where you have possibly neglected the value of spending more time or emphasis in any of these areas.

If initiating or committing to the cultivation of keystone habits is a new concept for you, then I encourage you to make a decision to develop these in your daily routine. These habits or changes in your daily behaviors are what will ultimately change your overall being and support your development of becoming the powerful leader and teacher you desire to be.

## Reflective Exercise

Journal your daily routine. How can you infuse the five keystone habits shared in this lesson into your action of service as a yoga teacher? Note where you see room to make small adjustments that will produce a larger impact as a yoga teacher.

# Developing a Highly Effective Teaching Methodology

"Teaching is more than imparting knowledge; it is inspiring change. Learning is more than absorbing facts; it is acquiring understanding."

— WILLIAM ARTHUR WARD

In this lesson, you'll step back and explore your overall approach to teaching while sharpening your awareness through the lens of five key areas that will support the development of a highly effective teaching methodology.

It's easy to shift our focus and efforts more heavily toward the technical aspect of our teaching skill set such as creating sequencing plans, curating our narrative, and theming our classes. These aspects of your teaching skill set are important and definitely have contributing factors in your ability to grow into a highly effective and skillful yoga teacher. However, let's pull back the lens and explore the viewpoint of your overall teaching methodology that encompasses much more than the technical competencies you'll need to develop.

Once you establish and lay the foundation of understanding upon knowing your role as a teacher, it's time to begin building upon that the framework of what will drive your overall intention and pursuits as a teacher. Once you have established this important element of teaching, then all other actions you will take within your teaching pursuits will continue to build from that acknowledgment and established methodology. Your teaching methodology will begin to reflect the type of teacher you desire to be. These two important understandings — role and methodology — will have a significant impact upon the impact and success you will have as a yoga teacher.

## The "How" Hunt

Oftentimes, we get caught up in desiring the "how" more than the "why" aspect of our pursuits. Getting caught up with the logistics of how you proceed along your teaching pathway before understanding the why that supports your overall quest will lead you on a never-ending, and possibly frustrating, "how hunt". This hunt will hinder your ability to make teaching yoga feasible and sustainable. The priority of action that is required to find sustaining success begins with a clear understanding of why you desire to teach yoga, however, oftentimes we place more focus on the need to know how that we end up finding ourselves in a continuous cycle of seeking to consume more when what is needed is to understand better why we're even doing what we're doing in the first place. The quest of consumption is a vicious cycle. In order to find sustaining success and fulfillment teaching yoga, the aspect of contribution will need to be factored in. If you focus more heavily on how or what you are going to do without first discovering and establishing the clear why that fuels your approach and teaching methodology, then you will quickly find yourself empty and burn out.

## Five Key Areas of Focus

In this section, I want to share with you five key areas that have contributed toward supporting continued effectiveness within my established teaching methodology as a yoga teacher. The points of focus that are highlighted ahead serve as great foundational bedrocks and directional markers to put into place to support the foundation of a highly effective teaching methodology.

## STUDENT-CENTERED

Let's begin with the student. This may seem obvious, because isn't the reason that someone decides to pursue teacher training to become a yoga teacher based upon the desire to share the practice with others? Well, I would like to say with one hundred percent confidence that this is the case, but it just isn't realistic. Unfortunately, sometimes rather than serving others as the intentional space behind why you're teaching, it can turn into a self-serving venture, instead.

Creating and establishing a student-centered teaching methodology will ensure that when you step into the classroom to lead and teach a practice, that your priority will rest in meeting the needs of the students where they are and within a learning environment that encourages a deep-dive exploration and encounter with the teachings of yoga.

You see, one pitfall of the ego that you can fall into if you're not aware and alert to it, is stepping in to teach as if you were the teachings. This teacher-centered approach suggests that the teachings of yoga come from you, rather than the teachings passing through you, which is a totally different approach and methodology. It's a matter of two words: from and through. A student-centered teaching methodology supports the bigger focus of being a teacher that passes the teachings freely along to others.

A student-centered methodology encourages deep thinking and guides and empowers others to create their own unique encounter in the practice of yoga with a deeper understanding of what the practice of yoga wants to teach us. This approach guides students beyond the surface of the exterior experience and beyond what the pose looks like or what is being produced. When your methodology resides and revolves around the student and their growth, you will teach and hold space from this same approach and method each and every time you step into the yoga classroom. This method equates to growth experienced mutually by the students and the teacher.

## MAKE CONNECTIONS

If your teaching methodology is student-centered then you will naturally begin to make connections. You will make interpersonal connections with students and begin to facilitate a space within the yoga practice where students can begin to connect the dots within the relational aspect of the yoga practice. Under your guidance, students will begin to make the cross-over connection between the experience they create on their yoga mats and the one they go out and create living their yoga off their mats in their daily lives. Become intentional about making these connections, keeping the practice focused within the student-centered approach so as not to create a disconnection where your focus is skewed and consumed with a self-serving agenda.

What can happen is that we begin to prepare classes believing that we know best what the student needs — and we can know, to a certain extent. However, there is also the space for listening that is involved within your methodology. Listen and respond to what you observe in the classes, what the students may be communicating, verbally and non-verbally as they interact with your directives and instructions during the practice. As you begin to observe more, you will pick up on how you can better support and meet the needs that are being communicated rather than solely what you assume is needed. When our methodology moves away from being centered around the student's experience, we begin to go into class and see the poses rather than the people, and this creates a barrier of disconnection.

## BUILD RELATIONSHIPS

As a yoga teacher, you cannot rely solely on the technical aspects of teaching. Teaching yoga is about building relationships, as well. Make engaging with students a priority. Students return to yoga classes because of the connections they experience and how you made them feel, not because they witness the expertise of a teacher on display. It is important to develop the technical aspect of teaching while balancing the relational aspect of teaching. When you balance the two aspects, you heighten the opportunity to nurture and nourish the soil of the yoga class experience. I've come to believe that this aspect is what brings students back to class.

## INCREASE INDEPENDENCE AND AUTONOMY

In order to be most effective within an approach that supports connection, we want to make sure the class experience is interesting and relevant for the students. This is where the language that we use to lead and guide the class makes a great impact on whether we will stay on the surface of the experience or allow our language to encourage others to pursue independence and autonomy.

The language and guiding cues that we use will either invite exploration and independence, or create dependence and subtle attachments that make students reliant on the teacher. Certainly, we want students to enjoy practicing with us but also being mindful that the greatest pursuit in teaching is one that guides others toward remembering for themselves so that they no longer need guidance from an external teacher. Focusing on supporting students in the development of autonomy within the practice experience is increased when students are provided space of independence and confidence in making choices that serve their practice needs. This approach and teaching methodology naturally gives permission for the freedom of choice to arise. This increase in autonomy arises from the teacher's willingness to release attachments to their agenda for the class experience and, ultimately, the prepared class sequence. We step into the classroom prepared in all of these aspects, yet, we empty ourselves of the plan so that we might step into the greatest gift we can give students: our presence.

## DISAPPOINTMENT: RED FLAG

It's important to note here that when you begin to notice that you are becoming disappointed when you aren't able to execute your planned sequence, this is a red flag that your teaching methodology is no longer student-centered. In fact, your teaching has become more about you fulfilling your agenda, and you are no longer seeing the students. You will know that your teaching methodology remains student-centered when you have prepared and equipped yourself to meet students where they are, adjusting your planned sequence accordingly, while staying committed to teach whoever walks into your class that given day.

Within this methodology, it's important to evaluate who you're planning for. Are you planning for the various students you will encounter? Or is your planned sequence based solely upon your preferences and abilities? Could you possibly be stepping in to teach and projecting your perceived experience upon the students, or are you open to the freedom of releasing and becoming empty of your plan? When we are rigid in our approach and teaching methodology, we are no longer student-centered. We become selfish. The evaluation then comes back to the inquiry of why you desire to teach.

## YOGA LITERACY

The last key area of focus to consider as you develop a highly effective teaching methodology is found within sharing and encouraging the development of yoga literacy. As yoga teachers, we must continuously pursue self-study. We find this within the aspect of remaining a student of the practice, even as we pursue the development of our teaching skills. Within self-study, yoga practice reveals to us what we lack knowledge of or do not see clearly. Whether it's our perspective that has been skewed from the attachment of our past experiences or the culture and conditioning of everyday life experiences, all humans struggle in these areas. Suffering comes in the form of attachments and delusion or, simply put, just not seeing clearly. This is the answer to why we practice yoga. It is the answer that Patanjali addresses within the ancient Yoga Sutras. We see this "problem" addressed from the very beginning of the Sutras, when the teachings of yoga begin to be shared and the dialogue and journey toward seeing more clearly through the applied practice of yoga is laid out before us. We also see that this condition of our minds has been present since the beginning of humanity.

So, why yoga? Well, why not? Because of the mental habits that continue to create suffering, the importance of a highly effective teaching methodology becomes evident if we are to support and provide students with a solution to this problem. We seek to equip students with the tools and applicable resources and practices they will need to first notice the habits. Then they can redirect their focus, realigning in a pattern of remembering that seeks an appropriate response rather than remaining in the cycle of reactive behavior that perpetuates more suffering.

Self-study will ask of you, as the teacher, to be in your own pursuit and quest to practice that which you teach. Increasing your yoga literacy, whether through the reading of wisdom texts, ancient and more modern, or through the application of the knowledge you are consuming is as important as the time you spend in the physicality of the asana practice. It is important that you are not only spending time within the physical practice of yoga asanas, but also challenging yourself in the mental preparedness that comes from being literate within the fullness of the yoga practice experience. This method supports you, as a student, and you as you lead and teach others about and within the practice. Take note that your effectiveness as a yoga teacher also resides in not leading others where you are not willing to go yourself. You will lessen your effectiveness when you try to teach from a place that you've memorized or read about but do not actually know from experience. There is a great vulnerability in self-study, but it will impact your ability to lead others along the journey with a genuineness and from a felt sense of knowing. It instills trust and increases connection, and it begins with dedication to your own pursuit of self-study.

Lastly, the yoga class setting is a co-created experience for you, as the teacher, to facilitate and hold space for others so that they can create the experience they wish to have. This space is vast, and it is inviting. The yoga classroom is a space that encourages exploration and independence. What type of teacher you will become is your choice. It begins with your teaching methodology. Understand where you are leading students and whether or not your current approach offers invitation and expansion. Or could you possibly be creating restrictions and limitations for students in their discovery process in the practice of yoga?

## Reflective Exercise

Write out your teaching methodology. Be specific. Why do you teach, and what is your primary focus and emphasis when you teach a yoga class? Reflect upon this often and evaluate whether it aligns and supports you in your ongoing pursuits as a yoga teacher.

# PART THREE:

# Leadership

# Introduction

To be a yoga teacher is to lead by example with quiet confidence, subtle humility, and grace. Mindset, motivation, and the application of "living your yoga" supports the ability to dive deep below the surface of teaching and it allows the teachings of yoga to flow from the essence of your heart so that, as a teacher, you become a conduit free and clear of distraction. The development of strong leadership skills as a yoga teacher resides within a balanced and developed teaching methodology. This encompasses strong technical competencies of teaching balanced with relational skills to support the ability to lead from a powerful place of identity, belonging, and transformation.

Leadership is reflected within the qualities of supplying motivation and optimizing engagement. The ability to lead by example comes through self-discipline and clarity. As you develop within the leadership aspect of teaching yoga, you begin to model, encourage, and inspire others to commit to the practice of yoga with the same disciplined behaviors. Strong and effective leadership empowers others and becomes less about managing or micromanaging. Within the development of strong leadership as a yoga teacher, we are able to not only lead the experience of the yoga class, but also equip others with the knowledge and experience of how to be a student of the practice.

"Who we are, is how we lead."
— BRENE BROWN, DARE TO LEAD

# Three Stages of Teaching

---

"Live as if you were to die tomorrow. Learn as if you
were to live forever."

**— MAHATMA GANDHI**

In this lesson, you will learn the three stages of teaching in order to better understand how to equip, apply, and take action
in your development as a yoga teacher. Learn how to create
a growth strategy and plan of action to apply what you have
already learned and determine when it's time to seek more
training.

The creation of a growth strategy plan will support you
within the various stages of teaching. Being a yoga teacher isn't a sprint. It is a marathon effort that requires you to
prepare, adapt, and adjust in order to maintain the pace and
growth that you desire to develop as a teacher. Becoming the
desired version of yourself as a teacher requires being with all
of the varied experiences and emotions that emerge along the
way and within the stages of teaching that I will share about
in this lesson.

Let's begin with the moments when you step out of yoga
teacher training. If you're reading and you have already experienced this, then take a quick moment to pause and reflect
back to your YTT experience. Depending upon how long ago
that was, can you remember the accomplishment you felt
when you received your completion certificate? And then did
you experience an unknown or possibly frightening emotion

of what to do next? Possibly, you wondered and questioned what your next steps would be. How were you going to now make this dream of being a yoga teacher a reality? Well, all of these emotions are certainly part of the first stage in your journey of actually taking action and teaching.

## Stage One: Transfer of Information

Let's dig a little deeper into understanding this first phase of teaching. It begins within the transfer of information. This initial stage begins while you are immersed and studying within your yoga teacher training experience, consuming and soaking up as much information as you can within this information transfer stage. Your lead trainer is conveying and sharing with you all that you will need to build a solid teaching foundation upon when you complete the training and hopefully providing you with all that you need to get started once you step out of the training. This is a crucial piece of the YTT experience, and part of the lead trainer's responsibilities, I believe, is to support and equip you well to go out to lead and teach in real time.

As a lead trainer of yoga teacher training programs, I always strive for this. In fact, it is a deal-breaker for me if trainees do not leave well-equipped with the tools to teach. Unfortunately and realistically, I know some of you reading may have not had that type of foundational YTT experience. And quite possibly, you completed the training but didn't feel equipped enough to teach. You might not have pursued teaching after the experience and left feeling like you needed to seek out yet another YTT to find the tools I've just described.

Trainees should leave their two-hundred-hour YTT with a solid teaching practicum base, meaning practice teaching was a large portion of the training curriculum. This includes the knowledge of how to apply and implement the structure of leading others though a yoga asana practice and leading from a level and high degree of understanding the intelligence behind sequencing and cueing. Nothing is random, so a foundational training should have a clear process and well-thought-out structure for how they train you to sequence and lead class practices. With this said, trainees also have a high degree of responsibility to show up, put in the work, and dedicate to this initial stage of learning and teaching. It is work. Just because you complete a YTT doesn't mean that you are good to go and that the learning ends. No, it means you have just begun, and you begin with what you know and what you have learned to get started. So start. Some of the best advice that I've ever received is that in order to get "better" at teaching, you must teach. So when you've taught a thousand classes, you know what? You teach a thousand more, as my teacher, Rolf Gates, instilled in me.

Confidence doesn't magically appear. It isn't handed out with your YTT completion certificate. You now must put into action what you know — and trust in what you do know, with faith so that you can begin implementing and applying the information that has been transferred to you. So you teach. This is the stage in which you will absorb and learn exponentially, and you will start to add layers onto the foundation that you laid during YTT.

As you gain experience teaching, you also gain confidence in yourself while developing the understanding that you are capable of being a yoga teacher. You know you have the capacity because it's already a certainty. It's something that you've already experienced and done before, so you know you are capable of doing it again. And again. It is the process, and this is the first stage of teaching.

## PURPOSE OVER PERFECTION

Will you step out of training and lead a yoga class perfectly? No. Will you get nervous, will you drop a pose or totally find your mind going blank at times as you try to recall which pose comes next? Sure you will. This is totally part of this initial stage of teaching. And let me tell you that even after more than two decades of teaching, I still get nervous at times as I step in to teach and lead a class. At times, I find myself not stepping in with what I like to call my "A-game" to teach. It's all a part of the ongoing process. Rather than perfection, it's about a continual commitment to the purpose and calling to teach. Part of the acknowledgment of this process is that it's also a reflection of being human. Students aren't coming to the classes you lead to encounter perfection; this doesn't exist. It's not realistic, and it's way too much pressure to heap upon yourself. In fact, this mindset can sabotage this wonderful learning phase that comes within this first stage of teaching. Students come to class to have an encounter, to develop a relationship. Students come to engage with presence, not only from you, but with the essence and relationship of the yoga practice that they are developing in their deeper understanding.

In this initial stage of teaching, be mindful that you aren't cultivating some type of desire for perfection as a teacher. Instead, your best efforts during this stage—and all stages of teaching really—are to dedicate yourself to the development of being fully present for the students you are guiding and leading within real time. Be mindful not to get distracted by an imaginary experience you've conjured in your mind while preparing to teach. Your undivided presence is a gift that you will impart to the students when they practice with you, and it's also a gift you will give yourself, because it will ground you and lead you to the next stage of teaching.

## STAY IN THE PROCESS

Just like the stages of being a yoga student, the stages of teaching reflect similar qualities. In this initial transfer-of-information stage, the act of doing becomes a prevalent piece. The application of the information being received is crucial for development. The actions we take within the practice and teaching come from having received details about the experience. There are a lot of details about the yoga pose shapes, including how to get in and out of the various poses, along with what to do while you're in the pose.

Early on in my practice, before I had even thought of teaching, and during this learning phase, I experienced an internal dialogue of questioning whether I was supposed to be inhaling, or exhaling, within the various actions and movement in and out of the flow sequence of postures. Eventually, I came to realize that, with dedication to consistency, it all came together naturally. The natural intuitive intelligence of the brilliance of my body's design began to guide me, and it was no longer about trying to intellectualize the process. Instead, I was harmoniously immersed with the natural rhythm of my body. This was a game changer, but it didn't come right away, and it's not always a harmonious experience that I have on my yoga mat either.

These details are important. As teachers, we initially learn a collection of cues to lead others into and out of the shapes, and hopefully, we do this skillfully and effectively with the guiding language we choose to use. We also hold space for students to figure this out on their own. There is no need to micromanage the process. We are guides. And as a guide, you respond and interact moment-by-moment to offer guidance that supports students to move independently through and within their bodies to facilitate a safe experience that reflects the natural intuitive intelligence of their body's design.

## TRUST THE PROCESS

It's always interesting for me, in the first weekends of yoga teacher training, how I find myself reminding trainees to be in the process of learning and to trust in the process. Trust in the process that has been designed for them to receive the information that I will be transferring to them. Usually, trainees are eager to learn — which is great — but with that, some are trying to get ahead of the process. I have spent many years designing and developing the training program curriculum that I follow in a way that layers the learning objectives and opportunities that I feel will best support trainees so that they leave my training program with a sense of knowing the information I'm sharing and transferring. I have had to put the brakes on some trainees over the years who come in with an attitude and belief that somehow they already possess this known experience of teaching for having practiced yoga for an extended period of time, or because they already possess certain aspects of a teaching skill set. Some come in feeling like the skill set they acquired as a yoga student will automatically transfer over into the act of teaching the practice, when, in fact, practicing yoga and teaching yoga require totally different skill sets.

What shows up quickly for most trainees I have taught is that guiding and instructing someone else through the practice experience seemed easy until they opened their mouths and attempted to led the group through a Sun Salutation series. Then what once felt, or seemed, easy became a paralyzing moment of not even knowing how to formulate the words, or directives, to lead this familiar sequence. I know this, so I incorporate learning objectives that support and equip trainees with tools to get started so that they can begin leading others as quickly as possible through practice teaching opportunities.

Let me share a little more from the student perspective when it comes to the transfer stage of teaching. Certainly, it is important that teachers remain dedicated students of the practice. However, there is an ongoing adjustment and evolving of the skill set that supports effective teaching. My goal as a teacher is to equip students with everything they need so that they no longer need my guidance. I certainly want students to practice with me, but my greater desire is that students aren't dependent upon me. This begins with the transfer of information.

Within this initial stage of teaching, information is presented, and the words used are mainly about the doing aspect of the practice. With time and dedication within this initial stage, we begin to slowly shift into the understanding of the layers beyond the physicality and our focus as students and teachers shift into the being aspect, or the somatic felt experience. The yoga asana provides us a vehicle for this exploration. It's important, as a student and as a teacher, that you give yourself time to be in the various stages of teaching so that you are steadily building upon your foundation without trying too quickly to get to the next stage. It requires an understanding of the process and developing trust in the process and in yourself. You will not step out of YTT and bypass the initial stage, because this would impede your ability to fully step into the next stages of your development and growth as a teacher. That requires patience. It is okay to be a new teacher. It's a beautiful space to reside in, so give yourself permission to be new and to grow in this new space.

## LEARN HOW TO BE A STUDENT

Oftentimes, our mindset shifts into a space where we somehow think when we venture into something new, that the transfer of information and the cultivation of this sense of knowing should happen automatically or in a short period of time. There is beauty and wonder to be found when we begin something new that requires us to give ourselves permission to be new and not know it all. Give yourself the opportunity to absorb and apply all of the information that has been transferred to you, and do so in your timing.

Along with trusting the process, you also need to be patient with the process. It's no different as a student. Beyond teaching the techniques of the practice, we are also teaching students how to be students of the practice. Ultimately, we teach others what we feel is important within the practice through how we communicate and instruct during the practice time, as well as, how we interact with students.

Within this initial stage of teaching, spend time evaluating the teaching experiences you have had and reflect upon what the students might actually be experiencing within the classes you lead. Set objectives for each class you teach and then make notes of reflection and points of feedback that support refinement and growth in your skill set. Seek to implement those mental markers you feel will support an impactful and effective learning experience for you and the students. Consider what students might actually be hearing from the cues and directives you use. If you aren't seeing the action implemented or the intended response from your cues, then seek to clean up your language. Lessen any confusion when it comes to what your intention is to highlight, and communicate with clarity throughout the practice session. This transitions nicely into the next stage of teaching.

## Stage Two: Personalize and Customize

You'll know you are shifting into the next stage of teaching when you begin to personalize and customize the instructions and cues you use to lead classes. In this stage, you begin to take ownership of your own teaching methodology rather than relying solely on the approach or script you learned in training. You'll begin to inquire into your own understanding more deeply rather than solely taking on the information that was transferred to you in YTT. This is the stage where you begin to investigate what you are saying and why you are saying it. You analyze and reflect upon your teaching experiences through a lens of refinement, gathering and gleaning information for the next time you teach. You also develop a willingness to refine and affirm to yourself again that you don't know it all and that is okay. You remain in the process of self-study and learning.

Years of experience teaching could lead one to feel like they have arrived at the end of their learning journey, yet, I have found I am now in a stage that is actually more about un-learning. It is about an acceptance that there is beauty in not arriving, not knowing it all. What fun would that be anyway? This perspective supports the beautiful mystery and pursuit that although teaching or practicing yoga is a quest, so to speak, it isn't about arriving or conquering. It is an experience that requires ongoing exploration and self-study. The space of curiosity remains in this stage of teaching, and learning, and unlearning, becomes an ongoing pursuit.

## NEXT TIME

Refinement is essential to becoming a highly effective yoga teacher. It will require those "next time moments" of evaluation. I incorporate these into the evaluation of every teaching opportunity I take part in.

Within this stage of teaching, you no longer rely on rote cues that supported you in the beginning, and you develop your own method of communication that includes a vocabulary of effective and guiding directives that fit your style of teaching. This doesn't mean you need to totally overhaul your cueing vocabulary, but you will begin to know what feels authentic and genuine to you as a teacher and quite possibly what you might start to say differently. This doesn't mean the cues presented during YTT aren't still relevant, but you must evaluate to remain effective. It is much easier to teach from a place you know and have had experience within rather than from a place you have memorized. This will always be the best place to teach from. This approach to cueing will equip you with quiet confidence when you step into the classroom. A good indicator that you're still in stage one is when you continually find yourself on your mat instead of out in the classroom, where you can connect more relationally and actually see the people you're leading, offering guidance beyond the physicality of the yoga pose.

Here's where the challenge to develop your skill set of teaching off your mat comes in. Trust me, I know it can seem or sound frightening in the beginning. I've been there. But I can also tell you with certainty that the moment I began stepping off my mat and trusting in what I did know without the need to demonstrate or "practice" with the students, then I began to expand and grow exponentially as a teacher. It was freedom, from being caught up in my head and to be among the flow of the class, facilitating an experience that becomes more about tapping into awareness of the present moment.

I will add here that discernment is always necessary when it comes to demonstrating. There is certainly a time when demonstrating a pose or transition is a key piece of the learning process for students. Your demonstration becomes an added layer of the learning process because what you might be instructing could be a new approach or unfamiliar. What I am referencing here is more about teachers feeling the need to be tethered to the mat. Thinking that your students need to see you is a myth. In fact, you may be staying on your mat because you lack confidence in yourself. Consider and discern when your need to stay on your mat and teach is more about a crutch, or hinderance, in your development as a teacher. And quite possibly, by remaining solely on your mat, you could be teaching students to become dependent upon the visual aspect of the practice. Evaluate all of this during this stage of teaching.

## PERSONALIZATION

The personalization aspect of this second stage of teaching supports the shift in developing the skill of seeing people rather than poses. This is where individualism merges with personalization—you being able to see individuals rather than the collective of the class. Your language shifts, and it's no longer about you directing with a one-size-fits-all cue. You no longer go in with a set sequence and become disappointed when you aren't able to teach what you had planned. You now step into the classroom, prepared and ready, yet you empty yourself of rigid attachment to a plan so that you can be present and open to the spontaneity of adjusting the plan to meet the needs of the students who are present with you in real time.

Within this stage, you broaden your approach. Your language begins to invite and encourage students to acknowledge their felt experience, guiding them to notice and feel. In this stage, you'll realize it's not about what you feel or your personal relationship with the practice. You choose not to project your experience on the students. Your personal practice experience helps to prepare you to teach, but you will choose language and cues that guide others to discover what they are experiencing rather than what you think they should be.

## Stage Three: Evolved Communication

The third stage of teaching begins to morph from the two other stages into an evolved means of communicating as a teacher. This evolution is evidenced in the way your words and language support the students' understanding and experience they encounter in the pose. A discovery is made by students through your effectiveness in the communication as they are invited to uncover and discover what has already existed within them all along. This becomes a driving factor behind the intention and teaching methodology that you carry into every class you lead.

This is it. The third stage of teaching becomes a stage where you no longer focus solely on creative sequences or teach from the same methodology and structure of sequencing each and every class. You can do this because of the work you've done in the other two stages. You aren't stepping into classes trying to reinvent the wheel, so to speak. Here is where freedom is expressed again. This approach and method for teaching will equate to growth not only for you, but also for the students you lead. Within this stage, you have repeatedly committed to absorbing and applying what you know; you have given yourself time to explore and refine. You commit to continual learning, and consuming more knowledge is no longer a distraction. You realize you have all you need in the moment to teach while still remaining faithful and committed to self-study and ongoing applied learning. By focusing on effective communication in a relevant, relational way, you lead students to see beyond the exterior shape of the yoga poses and encourage them to explore a fresh encounter within the interior of their experience. This way, they might transfer and carry the experience into their everyday living. This is what it means to live your yoga.

This stage and level of evolved communication supports students with an experience that reaches deeply into the body, mind, and psyche. Within this stage, your focus as a teacher has become more than just teaching techniques of the practice. This stage is all about touching the lives of students while serving and equipping them with all the tools of the practice that support their lives with the balance of ease and effort.

## Putting It All Together

Oftentimes, we dissect concepts so that we might learn and better understand what we are studying. As with other aspects of learning, it's important to take these dissected pieces of new understanding and fit them back together into the wholeness of experiential learning and come to know the topic or concept more fully. Through this deconstruction of key points and application, we begin to strengthen our foundation of understanding and develop applied wisdom. It is the same with teaching. It's important to note that the stages of teaching do not each stand alone. Throughout your ongoing pursuit and development as a yoga teacher, you will find yourself in a cycle of rotating through these stages throughout your career of teaching. Through the various teaching stages, you will continue to pursue in this quest of realization and discover the expanded version of yourself as a yoga teacher.

## Reflective Exercise

Journal about your personal stages of teaching. If you have not entered into a particular stage that was shared in this lesson, then envision what you desire that particular stage to be in your development as a yoga teacher. Begin now to create and develop a growth strategy for your teaching career.

LESSON 19:

# The Inadequacy of Information

---

"Our deepest fear is not that we are inadequate.
Our deepest fear is that we are powerful beyond
measure. It is our Light, not our Darkness, that most
frightens us."

— MARIANNE WILLIAMSON

Knowledge can be distracting. Consuming and accumulating knowledge without application can actually become a distraction and block development. In this lesson, uncover how the inadequacy of knowledge and information can create an insufficiency in your evolution as a teacher. Discover keys ways you can apply what you are learning and absorb knowledge as you teach what you need to learn.

You've probably heard the saying "knowledge is power," but is knowledge, in and of itself, really powerful? Piling on knowledge without application could actually become a barrier from growing and expanding your experience and perspective. Inadequacy equates to insufficiency. When we consume knowledge and never apply it, then we could be cultivating inadequacy, when, in fact, we just need to apply what we already know. We need to take a deep dive below the surface and spend time exploring the depths of wisdom that comes from absorbing and applying knowledge.

Within the yoga culture, it would seem there is a greater pursuit and quest for those who choose yoga teacher training. Yoga teacher trainings have become an industry. Many programs churn out high numbers of teacher trainees but spend very little time within the application or apprenticeship and mentorship of study that comes within the experiential aspect of teaching. Others provide and transfer a lot of information without much guidance about implementing and actually applying the concepts and information. No wonder so many trainees come out of training programs feeling insufficient, and some even seek additional training, as well as more information.

It is from the place of applied learning and absorption that we become equipped to share the teachings of yoga with others. There must be a time of refinement and molding that comes through the application of the knowledge we have received and the curating of confidence found within this space of knowing. Allowing the information to float on the surface will take you only so far within your pursuits as a teacher.

Deeper understanding involves internalizing a concept. It involves application. As you apply and prepare to teach, you must remain attentive and dedicated to your personal practice time. From your unique experience, you will begin to know better how to develop yourself as a teacher. Be sure you are looking within to find this deeper understanding rather than solely looking outside of yourself within the consumption of more knowledge. Get on your mat, and get on it often. Devote to this precious time and dig deeper into your understanding for yourself so that you'll become better equipped to share and lead someone else from a place that you know rather than a place you have intellectualized.

## Paralyzed by Information

We put so much of our resources—our time, money, and energy—toward the acquisition of knowledge that if this knowledge is not used, the overaccumulation begins to paralyze us from taking action. We find ourselves uncertain what to do with the knowledge we have, let alone the knowledge we layer upon. We become better consumers rather than more skillful and effective teachers. Knowledge is power, but time is money. The time and attention you give something is the true price you pay for it, but it doesn't always have to cost dollars. It could be your time and the application of gaining the power of the knowledge through application. Knowledge is power, but without action, it is useless. And you become a mere collector rather than a contributor.

## Application

Where do you start when it comes to applying the knowledge you've already acquired? It begins with the realization that you don't have to know it all to begin. In the context of teaching yoga, begin with what you do know from your personal experience of the yoga practice. Begin to build upon the knowledge and nuggets of wisdom shared and given to you by your teachers and others. If you're a new teacher, be a new teacher. Be in the learning process. Understand better the action of how we learn.

Consider this analogy, image you have a bucket and every time you try to fill this bucket, ninety percent of the water leaks out. You probably would not fill this bucket until the leak was fixed, right? Well, the same applies to all of the reading you do or the consumption of more knowledge. Your retention rate is going to be minimal if you do not address the absorption requirement that comes from the process of turning knowledge into applied wisdom, you will retain little. That's the leak in your bucket and this retention leak will diminish your capacity to pour into others effectively. Research has shown that people retain ninety percent when we teach someone else because we see the gaps in our knowledge instantly. Through the act of teaching, we can begin to understand where these gaps reside — where our bucket is leaking.

Even if the books you read and the lectures you listen to during YTT are very engaging, you will not retain much if you do not apply what you learned. Your interpretation of the concepts and teachings will always be different from that of the speaker, teacher, or author. There is a big difference between knowing something and understanding it. Knowledge becomes powerful and effective only when applied.

Begin to create opportunities to share the practice in a variety of ways to a variety of individuals. Consume less and make space for the time of deeper learning through application. If you keep piling on information, you will run out of space for the creativity of who you are to shine through as a teacher. When you create more than you consume, you will not only begin to create the teaching career you wish to have, but you will find success and fulfillment within the ongoing pursuit of refining and implementing the skills you already possess within you while exploring and applying the next layers of learning that will up-level your teaching skill set.

## Reflective Exercise

Take inventory of the teaching skills you feel proficient in. Evaluate the areas where there are "leaks" in your bucket and where you sense gaps. Evaluate where the gaps are located in your learning. Develop and create an action plan of how you will apply the knowledge you do have while continuing to study and absorb the knowledge that will enhance your development and growth as a teacher.

# Seasons of Being a Yoga Teacher

*"The teacher who is indeed wise does not bid you to enter the house of his wisdom but rather leads you to the threshold of your mind."*

— KHALIL GIBRAN

Look to nature and understand how to apply the cycle of seasons in your perspective of being a yoga teacher. In this lesson, you will look closely at the process of teaching from the start point to the closing of various teaching seasons, along with the transitional aspects found in between. Understand how to apply the seasons of teaching into your overall understanding and development of longevity as a yoga teacher.

## Start Point

Everyone has a start point. And you have possibly begun your journey toward becoming a yoga teacher already. Remaining a dedicated student is a key aspect of creating sustainability in what will be required of you as a teacher. Whether you are a new teacher or you've been teaching for a while, I want you to join me in reflection.

Somewhere along the way, you desired to learn and know more about the practice of yoga. Diving into a yoga teacher training isn't for everyone. There are other ways in which you can immerse yourself in the teachings and deeper study of yoga. The experience of YTT does provide a wonderful learning environment, and what better way to learn something more fully than to learn through the act of teaching someone else? Let's explore how this applies within the concept of seasons.

## New Beginnings

We can all relate to the season of a new beginning in our lives. This shows up, and we have most likely experienced this in a variety of ways. For the yoga teacher stepping out of teacher training, this is your start point. This is your new beginning. And just like other new beginnings that we encounter, we will also meet them with discomfort and even frustrations. The primitive area of our brain seeks comfort and security, and the idea of learning or experiencing something new sends signals, and sometimes red flags, that indicate this may not be a good idea. It doesn't feel comfortable. It is not a known experience from which we draw comfort, from where we feel secure in what we know. This space of new beginning feels foreign. It can even feel fearful. The primitive region of our brains will try to convince us that we shouldn't be pursuing whatever this new beginning might be. It's too hard. But life is hard, isn't it?

Once you step out, you begin. You must then resolve to seek consistency from dedication toward being in the uncomfortable space of the new beginning. You simply have to be where you are and in the process of the season you are in. Our brains once again will try to tell us to move on or paralyze us from taking action in this pursuit to gain experience learning and refining.

For the new yoga teacher, the learning season provides you with the opportunity to gain valuable insight and knowledge through the application that comes from real-time teaching experiences. Once you complete YTT, you are faced with a choice. Quickly, you encounter the reality of what will be required of you in order to make the dream and desire of being a yoga teacher a feasible ongoing pursuit. In this season, there will be quite a bit of effort involved as you gain momentum and traction teaching. This is where it might be helpful to liken this season of learning to the experience of the asana practice. Think back to the beginning of your yoga practice, the first time you stepped onto your yoga mat even. Just like practicing yoga brings a variety of emotions that we encounter—physically, mentally and spiritually—so does the act of teaching and the steady endurance that is developed and required to sustain this effort.

The beginning is not easy. It's filled with many unknowns. There is an adjustment period and encounters within the realistic understanding that practicing yoga and teaching yoga are entirely different skill sets. Teaching can feel exhausting and even lonely at times. But with all of that said, I want to reassure you that it is worth the commitment. Part of the responsibility of being a yoga teacher is to understand your capacity to support the work and stewardship of sharing the practice of yoga. In the beginning, there is an eagerness to teach. However, if you aren't observant, you will quickly find yourself teaching way too many classes and on your way to burnout and exhaustion due to being out of balance because your personal practice time has diminished. Your personal practice time is a gift—a gift given to yourself. This time supports your efforts and ability to teach; however, your personal practice time is not about preparing for your next class. This time is yours alone. This time is for you and not about giving to others. We cannot give to others that which we do not have to give.

Being a new yoga teacher is beautiful. Be okay with being new—and this applies to anything new in your life. Being new at something encourages us to continually seek to grow and refine through the act of learning.

## Becoming a Yoga Teacher

After twenty years of teaching experience, I found myself at a time, a season, of wondering what was next. From a deep desire to continue offering support and encouragement and to share my experiences of teaching with other yoga teachers, I created my Beyond Yoga Teacher Training Podcast, along with my mentorship program. The expansion of my teaching career now focuses heavily upon providing and equipping teachers with necessary resources that I know they will need to further their work of service in becoming the teachers they desire to be. I share this because I have first-hand experience and have come to know that there will be times in your career as a yoga teacher when you will need to evaluate and make decisions that support your ability to embody and become more fully present as a teacher. The season of becoming will be expressed in a variety of ways.

Within this evaluation—and the season of becoming—you will assess the balance that is present for you as a student and as a teacher. What you will quickly find as you begin pursuing the teaching pathway—and especially if you are doing so "full-time"—is that time management will be a factor. You'll need a strategy in place that supports your ability to adjust and figure out how to find the balance between your personal practice time and the time you are teaching others. Within the season of becoming, you are dedicated to the cultivation of confidence within your technical teaching skills while learning and growing through and from your real-time teaching experiences. You will want to tap into the intuitive space within you that notifies and signals you when you are out of balance, teaching more than that which supports your ability to remain faithful and dedicated to your personal practice time. If your personal practice time becomes nonexistent, then sound the alarm—this is a wake-up call. An adjustment is required and needs to be implemented quickly.

Manage your teaching time in a way that allows your personal practice time to remain a priority. If you continue trying to pour from an empty cup or a cup that is overflowing because you've got too many classes or trainings filling it up, then you are on a fast track to burnout. Within this acknowledgment, you will need a season to reset.

You may be wondering, though, how you can take this time of reset when you are trying to make a profession as a yoga teacher feasible and sustain your ability to generate an income that supports your daily living expenses. It sounds like reset means taking time off. For some, this will be the option that works best. For those who rely solely on teaching income, this may sound unattainable. In these circumstances, a teaching mentor, or coach, will be of great value as you seek to sift through your schedule and make the necessary changes that will redirect your focus. Analyze your time management so that you can select teaching positions that will support the balance.

## Priority of Action

A few years back, my family moved back to my hometown where my husband and I actually grew up, and it has been a wonderful transitional season in our life. This transitional season obviously began prior to our actual move, but none-theless, the move was a result of an acknowledgement and shift that set us up for the action that we would take for the move to take place. Within the moving process—because that was a process—I found myself forced really—I mean I had to—go through all of the stuff that had been accumulated and stored in a house that we had lived in for fifteen years. I have three boys, so there were closets and storage areas where we had stored a lot of stuff. This transitional season asked me—very abruptly, I might add—to get organized and make some decisions on what was truly necessary and of priority to make the move into our next home and into the next season of our lives.

It's the same concept for you as a yoga teacher. When you intuitively notice and feel that you are out of balance—and I do believe this is a felt experience—you must, first of all, ac-knowledge it. Acknowledge the reality of the process you're currently in and then discern and make decisions that will support your ability to realign, reset, and rest to fill yourself again with the passion that you first encountered when you began the practice of yoga. Evaluate your schedule and clean out some closets, so to speak. Notice where you are efficient with your time and where you might need to make decisions that support your capacity to "work smarter, not harder." Get creative and use the knowledge you already have to create a fresh encounter for yourself as a student and then as a teacher.

If you ignore this season in life, chances are you will find yourself stuck in a rut and your brain will tell you again that this is hard or that there's no way out. Your brain might even tell you that it's not worth the effort, and you need to quit. My advice in these moments, these seasons, is to get still. Get still so you can listen. You could say it's time to go back to the beginning. Tap in to the space that drew you to your yoga mat in the beginning. It's important to note here that this season may require you to actually take some time away from teaching. It may require you to make a hard decision to relinquish your teaching responsibilities during this season of reset and realignment. It may require you to retreat, find respite, and refuel.

Refuel yourself by reallocating the time toward your personal practice. Your mat is where inspiration and creativity resides for you as a student and teacher. If left unattended, though, the priority of your personal practice time can become neglected.

## Season of Reflection

Found within the season of becoming is reflection. By this time, you have most likely accumulated many teaching experiences to reflect upon. In this season, you re-evaluate your reason for teaching and why you're doing what you're doing. You evaluate why you are continuing to pursue the path you're on as a teacher. Reflect on whether you are stuck in a rut. Is it time to make a detour and explore another path? Possibly, it is. Spending time reconnecting with the passion and purpose from which you were first called is a continual investment of time and reflection. It is a well-made investment. This reflective season will support your ability to sustain longevity in this work of service. I also want to encourage you to affirm yourself that when you do take the time to reset and potentially step back from your teaching responsibilities that it does not mean that you are no longer a yoga teacher. Just because you aren't teaching a scheduled class on a regular basis does not mean that you are no longer a teacher. What has happened is that the role has shifted, and another layer of the role of yoga teacher has emerged for a season. All that you have invested in and gained through the act of teaching has not been diminished. During this season when you may not be active teaching asana, that doesn't mean you aren't still invested in the ongoing pursuit to know the various facets of the practice more deeply. From my experience, this time of reset is just what was needed in order for me to step back into teaching refreshed, renewed and ready to teach and share the practice of yoga with others.

## Season of Experience

This leads to the season when teachers find themselves having taught for an extended period of time. This season is about what is done with all that has been experienced and learned. The birth of my podcast and mentoring program came at a time when I was in deep reflection, finding myself with two decades' worth of teaching experience. I asked myself, "What now?" For me, my teaching path is driven from the continual relational aspect of teaching and the pursuit, first and foremost, to know the practice more intimately for myself.

Experience has taught me there is a natural byproduct that spills into my ability to lead, connect, and share the practice with others more fully because of this investment. This is where the ease shows up. Today, there is less effort when it comes to teaching. Sequence preparation, what to say and how to cue, starts and resides in the beautiful space that I know, and that's the space I share from. I remain in constant refinement of all of the technical aspects of teaching because it is important and contributes greatly toward our ability as teachers to connect others to something much bigger.

## Beauty in Not Arriving

One could say that the experienced yoga teacher has arrived. Quite possibly, there is a beauty to be found in not arriving, not knowing it all. It's the beauty that we find in the seasons of nature that teaches the timing of all things — the time to enjoy and be with life as it is, the time to embrace change, and the time to move on, allowing one season to end so that a new one might begin. If you have been teaching for a while, then you're a seasoned yoga teacher, and I challenge you to stay the course, continue to invest in yourself, and be willing to learn and explore new understandings within your relationship with the practice of yoga.

## Reflective Exercise

Take a few moments to journal how you see the cycle of seasons — beginning, becoming, and reflecting — represented within your teaching path. Consider the transitional times between these seasons in your time of reflection. Consider the emotions that seasons bring and the plans you'll make to support you within and throughout the various seasons.

# Mindset Matters

"Tools of empowerment—heartset and mindset."
**– AKOSUA DARDAINE EDWARDS**

In this lesson, learn the qualities of a growth mindset and how it will set you up for success, growth, and development, as an individual and as an effective yoga teacher. The evaluations of how and why the thoughts, stories, and dialogues that we habitually have throughout our days really do matter. It matters because what begins as a thought in our minds will ultimately lead to the actions, and inactions, that we will take in our everyday life.

I think we can all agree that, as humans, we are all easily distracted. And if we aren't aware and intentional about the distractions that derail our everyday living, then we will quickly find that we are floating through life, missing out on the interactions and encounters that make life so sweet and enjoyable. Advancements in technology have been great; however, they have also become subtle, numbing distractions that take us out of the genuine and authentic experiences of connected life experiences. Digital distractions can quickly lead you to fall into the comparison trap and into the world of feeling like you're living life as an imposter.

I recently was traveling from North Carolina to Montana, and it required flying, which then required some layover time in between flights. You can most likely relate to this not-so-fun aspect of airline travel. I knew there would be a lot of effort in the process of getting to and from where I was going. This "process," the relatively short time of uncomfortable travel within a layover was going to be required, was well worth the effort because it ultimately lead me to my desired destination and, more importantly, a wonderful time watching my oldest son play baseball. I really do enjoy traveling, and when planning this trip, I made many of my decisions based upon the cost-saving aspect. That meant choosing flights that were anything but convenient and that my flight would be comprised of not one, but two stops. In my decision-making and planning, I knew that there would be a significant effort made to arrive at our destination. Once again, this "effort" was going to be well worth it and would help us accomplish our ultimate goal and desire for taking the trip in the first place.

I share this travel story because it pairs nicely as we proceed into this lesson regarding mindset. I love how the imagery of travel is relevant and correlates to life's enduring and sometimes lengthy journey. And when we think of the yoga practice and how often we hear it described as being a journey, it helps us to better understand the process and how our mindset impacts our ability to trust in and stay in the process, because ultimately, the journey is our destination.

## The Space of Waiting

Distractions can intrude and impact the thoughts and stories that we play over and over within our minds daily. Going back to my airport story—as we waited during one of our layovers, a four-hour layover, I found myself sitting at the gate, awaiting my next flight. During this time, I thought I would be productive and catch up on emails and social media posting. During this time, I remember taking a pause, and in a clear moment of awareness of the space I was in, I looked up from my distraction. What I quickly noticed was that everyone around me, from as far as I could see, had their heads down, staring into a screen. Now, isn't this a reflection of our daily lives? I wondered, was everyone in that airport space seeking a distraction from the inevitable experience that we were all collectively having at that time? Were we all seeking a distraction from having to wait? No one likes waiting, right? We are a society that has everything at our fingertips, so why should we ever have to wait on something or put any effort toward waiting for what we desire.

I'm not sure that any of us can say that we enjoy layovers in airports, but it makes me wonder how much of life we are choosing to be consumed within our minds, distracted from the moment or space we are actually in, the space of presence. It really does require effort and continual reminders to be present, to be where our feet are. Yet, the plight and trickiness of our minds tells us differently. The mind, if left untethered, is scattered and distracted. And possibly we have no idea where we really are or where we're even trying to go. We are in a state of "hovering," as I like to call it. We are waiting to put down our landing gear and get grounded. Here's where the wonderful practice of yoga comes in. It is a practice that supports our ability and capacity to land—to anchor into the present moment by tethering our mind to our breath and awareness.

## Why Mindset Matters

Your mindset is a set of beliefs that shape how you make sense of the world and yourself. It influences how you think, feel, and behave in any given situation. Let's explore the development of a mindset that is oriented for growth and expansion so that you might begin to enjoy where you are and be fueled for your travels as you make your way through all of the wonder and beauty on this journey we call life.

Let me ask you this—could your mindset, your thoughts and beliefs of yourself have an impact on your ability to be successful? Yes, and research suggests your beliefs and what you are thinking play a pivotal role in what you want out of life, in life experiences, and in whether you achieve those wants and desires.

## The Fixed Mindset and the Growth Mindset

To better understand the broad strokes of mindset, there are two basic categories to consider: (1) fixed mindset and (2) growth mindset. A fixed mindset believes that one's abilities are fixed and unchangeable. A fixed mindset can also believe that talent and intellect is all that is needed, without any effort. In contrast, a growth mindset believes that talents and abilities can be developed over time with effort and that everyone is capable, to some degree, of becoming more knowledgeable and talented if effort is placed behind that desire.

Research suggests that our mindset is developed early through praise and labels and the mindset developed will vary dependent upon the type of praise we received. For example, personal praise given toward a particular talent or being labeled "smart" in childhood promotes a fixed mindset. The message sent early is one that suggests that either you have an ability or not and that there is no changing that. The idea of "process praise," however, emphasizes the effort and accomplishments in achieving a task. This implies that success is due to effort and strategy, both of which can be controlled and improved upon over time. It's important to understand that by focusing on the process rather than the outcome, we can better understand that our efforts, hard work, and dedication can lead to change, learning, and growth both now and going forward.

I'm pretty sure you've heard the phrase "trust the process." I use this quite often when I lead teacher trainings. Often, we miss what's taking place, along with the learning opportunity, while we are actually in the process of obtaining the desired result or achievement we seek because we are more focused on the actual end result or desired outcome. We are often frustrated when we want to begin something new and assume we should learn quickly. That just isn't a guarantee, though.

I believe that trainees often step into the training experience without fully realizing there is a process that consists of the exchange of information, the application of the information being shared, and the ongoing absorption of information and knowledge. And time is a big factor in this process, as well. Realistically, we cannot set a time, or deadline, on when the absorption will take place. Completing a yoga teacher training doesn't mean you will magically, or instantly, be all that you desire to be as a teacher. It doesn't work like that.

## Commit to the Long Haul

Yoga teacher training is a start point, a place of discovery, where all that you are capable of and all that you hopefully will aspire to be is fuel for the ongoing learning pursuit and quest that comes with teaching and leading others through the practice of yoga. From my experience, you should ask yourself whether you are committed to the long haul of the journey of being a yoga teacher. Are you willing to be in the process and all that the process has to teach you along the way?

I also believe when it comes to the development of a growth mindset that it's important to trust in what you do know at any given time and understand that devotion and dedication to the process will lead you toward that ultimate success in whatever you are pursuing as a teacher or as an individual. I'll emphasize here, too, that I am being vague and broad with the term success because that can be interpreted in a variety of ways according to each individual, and I am intentionally using it within that context. It's the same with the students you lead. You're number-one priority is that students are successful according to their own terms and what they seek and aspire to achieve within the yoga practice.

Understanding the layers behind the development of your mindset is vital for your success in anything that you do in life. Your mindset will make a big impact on your ability to create longevity as a yoga teacher. A lot of backend work has to take place to prepare you to be effective and skillful as a teacher, and this goes well beyond being prepared with the technical aspect of delivering a sequence of yoga poses. Although that is certainly important, it isn't everything when it comes to teaching. In order to sustain and create longevity teaching, you will be challenged and required to rely on much more than your technical skill set as a teacher.

At some point in your teaching journey, you will need to pause, reflect, and investigate the layers of requirements for teaching that go beyond teaching the poses. Interestingly, there isn't a lot of time or focus placed on this topic in yoga teacher training. That's why teacher training is merely a start point. It's kind of like the yoga practice and asana. The asana gets your attention. It is what is seen, what we relate to externally. It is the start of the exploration of discovery. And this is the same for the yoga teacher.

Initial teacher trainings or the two-hundred-hour foundational trainings are just that—a foundation. Upon that you will build with effort—and sustaining effort, I'll add.

When I lead two-hundred-hour yoga teacher trainings, it is my intention that those who train under my guidance know how to lead an asana class and how to do so effectively and skillfully with a deep understanding of the reasoning and intention behind what they are leading. Remember, asana is the start point in most of our lives and the experience with yoga, so if you are going to be a yoga teacher, you need to be well-equipped to lead a class experience that supports success in the development of the various layers that will be built upon that initial foundation and understanding of the practice of yoga.

## Student-Focused Mindset

Consider all that I've just shared as layers of support in the cultivation of a teacher's growth mindset that is student focused and aligned within an overall focus of the success that you desire for each and every student you share the practice of yoga with. Let's discuss more about your teaching emphasis and how that will correlate directly with forming a growth mindset.

Let's begin with intention. What intention are you setting for the students you lead, and what are you communicating beyond the cues and technical aspect of the yoga class sequence? Your role is to reflect back that which is already in existence within every student. Reflect back the inherent wisdom that is already within each individual and trust that

SANDY RAPER

students are capable of remembering and knowing this space of wisdom. A student-focused growth mindset will seek first to meet students where they are and then discern how to facilitate the best experience that provides success for each student.

## Mindset Evaluation

I'll conclude with sharing a couple of suggestions that will support you in the development of a growth mindset. If you feel like you already operate within a growth mindset, then use these suggestions to support you further within evaluation processes.

First, focus on the journey. There's that metaphor again. It's not about the destination, which is where we often get caught up; it's about all that we experience, learn, and come to know along the way. All life experiences have something to teach us. Perhaps when you focus on the journey, you'll actually find yourself somewhere along the path that is far better and expansive than you had limited yourself to believe in. Trust the process of the journey.

Secondly, incorporate the word *yet* into your vocabulary and conversations with yourself. If you're struggling, remind yourself that it's okay to not know something or to have not mastered a skill… *yet*. Incorporating this word encourages and supports you during and through the struggles and obstacles that come with learning something new. Anything new and worth pursuing is going to present obstacles, and a growth mindset will seek to learn and grow even through what might initially feel like a struggle or setback. Consider what every experience in life can potentially teach you rather than allowing circumstances to become a tormenter. Isn't that really why we practice yoga? We practice to notice and acknowledge the habits of our mind that create suffering in our lives. We seek to remember the practices of yoga that are available to align us back into the space of a life, awake and present.

Thirdly, pay attention to your words and thoughts. What you say matters — it matters what you say to others and what you say to yourself. Reverse and replace negative thoughts with thoughts that are positive, nurturing and initiate growth.

Lastly, embrace and take on challenges. You will learn through all experiences, even the ones we deem mistakes. Be courageous and put yourself out there. Learn something new, and trust the process along the way. You might have a layover toward your ultimate destination, and you might even find yourself on a detour. Regardless of which it is, trust in the process that will guide you to your ultimate destination.

## Reflective Exercise

Take some time to journal these prompts. (1) Do I have a fixed mindset or a growth mindset? (2) Do I believe that I am capable of changing my mindset? (3) Do I believe that others have the same capacity?

# Teaching from Intuitive Intelligence

---

"Intuitive guidance, however, is all about change. It is
energetic data ripe with the potential to influence
the rest of the world."

– CAROLINE MYSS

In this lesson, delve into the concept of how to apply the
knowledge received during your yoga teacher training and
develop the ability to teach by "reading the energy of the
room." You can develop the ability to step into each yoga class
with an immediate understanding and knowledge of how to
lead a skillful, supportive and effective yoga class with intuitive intelligence rather than analytical or intellectual reasoning.

## Reading into the Energy of the Room

An important skill set to develop as a yoga teacher is one that
goes beyond the technical aspect of teaching. The concept of
reading into the energy of the room expands into the relational aspect of teaching and is a developed skill that will support
you in discerning quickly the information you are gathering
so that you can provide optimal guidance to support the students. In order to provide context and support in understanding this concept further, we'll first dig into the meaning of the
term intuitive intelligence.

Intuition is an immediate understanding, or knowing, of
something without reasoning. By reading the energy of the

room, you can actually begin to develop the ability to step into the yoga class you are leading, any class, and meet the students where they are, understanding what they need and adapting and adjusting any asana practice to meet those needs. It means you step in without overanalyzing, micromanaging, or trying to make reason out of needing to make the class sequence you planned fit even if it doesn't serve or support the students who actually showed up for class that day.

It's important to understand that the methodology, or approach, of reading energy is a skill that can be developed, and it's best developed within the real-time experiences of teaching. Application is a vital piece of your overall development and growth as a teacher, and it will give way to the building of other aspects of teaching, such as confidence. It's beyond your YTT experience that the responsibility shifts from your lead teacher trainer to you.

As you begin teaching and applying what you learned in training, your responsibility shifts to the next developmental aspect of being a teacher. It becomes a time of taking on responsibility for your own development rather than sitting back and choosing to replicate what you learned from the lead trainer or your favorite yoga teacher. Your responsibility now is to discover that aspect of yourself, and you do this through the act of teaching. During this season, you will teach and begin to build trust in yourself through the process of being in all of the developmental stages of teaching. This concept requires effort, but with time and application toward this approach to teaching, you will begin to experience ease.

## Developing Intuitive Intelligence

There is also an instinctual element that supports the cultivation of the concept of reading into the energy of the room. Teaching from this space of immediate knowing and understanding of what is needed in the real-time yoga practice experience offers a sense of freedom that gives way to trust and confidence because you also trust in your intuitive capacity to apply this teaching approach every time you teach.

When I developed this leadership aspect and approach to teaching, the mysterious doubt began to dissipate. I trusted in my abilities because I had been there before. I knew I was capable. I continue to step into every class, into every training and workshop I lead, with this same confidence and intuitive intelligence.

Confidence is developed within the embodiment of your applied experience. Intuitive intelligence is no different. It is a matter of having a plan and then being willing to relinquish the plan when you step into the class to teach. You relinquish the attachment to your plan, becoming empty so that you might better serve those you are leading. If you are filled with attachment or rigidity to your plan, then you lessen the opportunity for students to see beyond the technical aspect of the practice. When you become empty and access the intuitive and instinctual aspect of your teaching skill set, you open up the class experience to be lead from intuitive intelligence and the bigger transformational working of the practice of yoga.

Each class I lead, I know that I am capable to lead and support the class experience within this approach. I confidently know that I can support the classroom in whatever capacity it needs or asks of me. I present myself in the room in a way that avoids getting caught up in my head, that space where we can quickly become entangled in the weeds of doubt, uncertainty and memorization. Instead, I choose to show up and intentionally empty myself of the structure and plan of the class. I am then able to sense and read the energy of the room. I discern. I adapt, and I choose to remain in that space for the duration of the entire class experience. I then repeat the process the next time I step in to teach and lead a yoga practice experience. Found within the repetition of this approach, ease is present and underpins the foundation of remembering that I am capable of leading from intuitive intelligence.

The class experience does not hinge upon a perfectly executed sequence plan, rather, there is a profound creation of a collective experience taking place in the present, and you can then trust that each student is successful in whatever way they might define success in their practice experience.

This type of teaching methodology allows for a powerful emergence of autonomy for students. And although I am leading and guiding through a collective class experience, students still find their own unique experience because the subtle trust that is present gives them permission to do so. As a teacher, you can hold that space for students — the space for them to encounter and develop autonomy all while keeping a watchful eye upon how you might better support the various needs within the ongoing class experience.

## Instinct

Within the development of your intuitive intelligence as it applies to your teaching methodology, instinct is present. This is where your subconscious and conscious regions of your brain begin to work together. It's where the instinctual brainstem region of your brain and the intuitive right-side region, the hippocampus, along with your "gut" come together in a collaborative effort. This aspect is where you are trusting your gut, along with your instinctual impulses and behaviors to initiate action holistically—and quickly. Actions are taken innately rather than remaining within the region of mental processing of information.

Our minds are wired to see patterns. Our brains not only process information but also store insights from our past experiences. Your intuition draws from this deep memory well and has been developing and operating since you were born. When we subconsciously spot these patterns, our bodies respond by sending neurochemicals to our brains and guts. These somatic markers are what gives us that instant insight into what feels accurate, appropriate even, or the opposite of what might feel off.

Since each person's intuition is based upon a collection of individual experiences, it is then also subject to opinion and bias. This is where it's important that you are exploring and choosing to be open to understanding and appreciating value in the thoughts and experiences of others. Couple this understanding with empathy in order to observe and discern how you might offer instruction and guidance from what you are bearing witness to as you evaluate how your cues and directives are impacting the students responses. All of this better supports the developed teaching methodology of reading into the energy of the room.

Consider whether or not you are open to students exploring their own unique experience of the asana practice rather than controlling the experience by projecting what you have experienced in the practice. This is where the language that we use to lead comes into careful consideration. As teachers, be mindful that your language isn't projecting what students should be experiencing. This projection diminishes the student's own development of autonomy and intuitive intelligence. Rather, consider guiding language that leads and directs students with curiosity and awareness of the experience they are creating.

Instead of telling students where they should be feeling an action within the asana, invite them to notice the targeted area and evaluate where their attention is being drawn in the given shape or movement. Support and equip students with the tools to connect the dots while they further explore and excavate the landscape of their practice experience.

The space of intuitive intelligence empowers us, as teachers, as well as the students we lead. This empowerment comes within the zone of ambiguity and change, which is also the space where imagination and genius occur. Intuitive intelligence becomes the space of immediate knowing and understanding. You begin to know this space more fully by initiating and acting upon the trust you have in yourself and the acknowledgment of this inner knowing and that you are, indeed, capable of remembering this aspect. As yoga teachers, we cannot rely solely on our technical competencies and skills to truly develop and grow in our effectiveness as teachers. It's just not that cut and dry, because we are working within the human condition.

## Cultivating Intuitive Intelligence

Intuition is also an immediate form of knowledge in which the knower is directly acquainted with the object of knowledge. Intuition is also currently understood to be the subliminal processing of information that is far more complex than rational thought. The processes that make up intuition are learned, not innate. Comparatively, instinct is not a feeling, but rather an innate, hardwired tendency toward a particular behavior.

## Knowing Yourself

Get to know the space of your intuitive intelligence for yourself. Get still, meditate, and explore within your personal practice time. Explore intuition when you move in and out of the various yoga postures. Inquire into where your natural intelligence and tendencies of your body's movements are leading you. What is your body communicating and inviting your mind to bear witness to beyond the analytical, or even critical, lens of analysis that can show up when we begin to observe and get to know ourselves more intimately. Notice when the mind begins to label and organize the experience. Notice when thoughts arise to judge the sensations or the experience you are having. Remember the patterns your mind seeks to create, as well as the stories around the experience in efforts to stay occupied or possibly distracted from what is actually taking place in real time. Perhaps it isn't a state of being occupied or entertained that the mind is seeking most. Perhaps it's the opposite. What if it was less about getting through the experience and more about being with the experience you are currently encountering? Perhaps the learning is to be found within the experience that is void of comfort, expectation, and assumption. Take time to explore this for yourself.

## Recommit to Your Personal Practice

Consider the current relationship you have with your yoga practice. I encourage you to rededicate to this time without any attachment of practicing in order to share or teach others. If you aren't careful, as a teacher, you can fall into the trap of thinking that you are dedicating to your personal practice yet what you really are doing is using your practice time to prepare to teach.

I challenge you to rewire your approach to your personal practice. Get on your mat, sit on your meditation cushion, and simply explore the practice for yourself. That's it. Redirect your thoughts away from the thinking mind that will use this time to plan and curate class sequences. Choose to approach your personal practice time within and through the lens of excitement for exploring a fresh encounter within the experience that is solely for your benefit. Journal or make small notes of the experiences you have on your mat.

## Trust Yourself

Trust in what you know. Trust in what you are learning and the experiences you are creating as you develop in your effectiveness as a teacher. This is where wisdom emerges. Acquire knowledge, in moderation, so that you can balance the acquisition with the action of application so that the knowledge might morph into applied knowledge or wisdom.

Being ready is about being prepared. When you are dedicated to applying the knowledge you gained, it prepares and supports your ability to cultivate and tap into your innate wisdom. This innate wisdom will prepare and equip you to take action so that you aren't waiting to be ready. Piling on knowledge, for knowledge's sake, without incorporating an ongoing process of application will not fill you up. Instead, this approach will leave you feeling empty and hinder you from stepping out to teach from what you already have, what you already know.

Lastly, what I have found to be true is that the development of intuitive intelligence resides within knowing you have a solid foundational plan for sequencing. This foundation is a key requirement for intuitive intelligence to be supported and developed. You will benefit greatly in your organizational plan of knowing why you are linking particular yoga postures together. Beyond the creative aspect of sequencing, there is a thoughtful and intelligent process for organizing asanas together within a skilled method that facilitates, supports, and invites students to move through and in their bodies in a way that sets them up for the creation of an experience that encounters success.

Your sequencing structure and plan includes movements that prepare the body physically, as well as, supports a concentrated effort of sustained attention for the mind. This provides students with the best opportunity to encounter awareness of the present moment found in the endurance of sustained effort while also finding ease within the entirety of the practice session.

Your approach to sequencing will indicate whether this created experience is feasible. Within this student-centered approach, you will know and trust that you leading students safely and creating an effective learning environment. You will begin to lead and teach from the space of intuitive intelligence when you are confident and solid in your understanding of the impact of sequencing and the why behind the method. From this solid understanding and foundation, you will then go in to lead and teach the same way, within the same method, each and every time you step into the yoga classroom. This approach leads to growth. Growth for you as a teacher and growth for the students you lead.

Teaching from the approach of reading the energy of the room supports a learning environment where students feel seen. Begin to better understand what the various shapes represent within a bigger context. See the beauty of autonomy reflected back to you, understanding that it's less about perfection or performance. As you step in to lead from this perspective and intention, students will join in with the same collective intention and emphasis for why they are practicing.

Teaching from intuitive intelligence equates to connection. This is where the powerful transformative qualities arise and become accessible within the practice experience. As a teacher, you support students in their abilities to notice, engage with, and practice the experience of tapping into their own intuitive and instinctual intelligence, as well.

## Reflective Exercise

Evaluate how confident you are in your sequencing structure. Write out your framework and make notes for how you will offer options and transitions between the various yoga poses. Take time to create mini-sequences of three postures and fit them together within the overall framework of your sequence. Practice teaching these sequences repetitively until you are confident in them and know how to adjust them to meet the needs of various student approaches within your class.

Trusting your intuition is all about trusting in yourself. Trust yourself as a student, trust the teacher who is guiding you, and ultimately trust the great teacher who resides within you. The more trust you place in yourself, the more success you will experience.

LESSON 23:

# The Biggest Obstacle for a Yoga Teacher

---

"At the end of the day, it's not about what you have or even what you've accomplished... It's about who you've lifted up, who you've made better. It's about what you've given back."

— DENZEL WASHINGTON

In the end, it's not about you. Teaching yoga is an act of service, where you ultimately fade into the background of the yoga class experience and allow the teachings of yoga to flow freely. In this lesson, you will learn how the quiet inner knowledge that you are capable of leading an impactful yoga class experience empowers others to pursue their quest and journey through the practice of yoga.

When it comes to confidence, it isn't about superiority or arrogance. In fact, it's quite the opposite. Someone who exudes the essence of confidence operates from a quiet inner knowledge that they are capable. The biggest obstacle that I have come to realize and I hear repeatedly from yoga teachers is a lack of confidence. In this lesson, you'll explore and uncover why this is and why yoga teachers continuously feel this way. We'll explore how to shift this belief so that you can become empowered to go out and serve your community by teaching yoga with true confidence.

## Confidence

Historically, confidence was thought of as an innate personal trait, something that you either were or were not born with. However, recent research has provided us with evidence that confidence can be learned and developed. Could it then be considered that yoga teachers are not confident because they haven't yet learned or developed this skill? From the definition and research I've already shared, you can find encouragement in knowing that confidence can be cultivated.

For many, the simple act of teaching will build a lot of confidence. But that is not the only piece of the development process. If true confidence is a feeling of self-assuredness that is grounded in an authentic experience of one's own ability, perspective, and sufficiency, then it's safe to say that in order for true confidence to emerge, you'll also need to fully embrace and acknowledge confidence in not only your teaching experiences but also how and what you are actually teaching.

This is where I believe this persistent obstacle of the lack of confidence lies for yoga teachers. Being hesitant about what you are teaching impacts how you teach. Begin by asking yourself if you feel grounded in a deep understanding of how to lead an effective, skillfully crafted yoga asana class experience. Being confident is a stable connection, and if you're lacking in confidence, then there is some type of disruption or instability. In this lesson, I will share some valuable, relevant, and actionable information that will support you in establishing a grounded connection that will allow you to develop and sustain confidence in yourself as a yoga teacher.

At times, the concept of confidence can seem vague, and you may find it hard to verbalize how it really applies to you and how you feel. I'm pretty sure you can recognize confidence in someone else when you see it.

Confidence is not only a feeling but also an experience. Therefore, you know when you are surrounded by confidence. In fact, confidence is a collective experience that is felt by not only you but others feel it, too. If confidence can be sensed and felt, then we can also associate an energetic quality with it. Within this recognition, this magnetic quality will draw other confident people to you.

## Confidence Teaching Yoga

If confidence has a magnetic quality, then it's important to note the impact that a confident yoga teacher can make within and on the overall practice experience. It can impact the quality of the class. If confidence can be felt and recognized, it would also imply that this state of being confident will take on some recognizable traits that you can begin to see when confidence is present. If we conclude that confidence is a felt experience, we can also conclude that we also sense insecurity. In the presence of an insecure person or even a person pretending to be confident, faking it until they make it, we not only notice their lack of confidence, but also begin to notice their attempts to compensate for it.

Interestingly, too, when we're in the presence of a self-doubting person, we often tend to feel self-conscious as well. There's that collective-experience piece again. We then struggle to connect organically and begin second-guessing our choice, noticing feelings of unease and uncertainty, which creates a disconnected experience. That is the opposite of the intention we set as teachers when we go in to lead classes. Our intention to serve others while connecting them with the teachings of yoga becomes unclear in the midst of a lack of confidence and it diminishes our leadership.

## Hurdle the Obstacle

The need, or requirement even, to hurdle this great obstacle in your path as a yoga teacher is vital. If you desire to lead and teach meaningful and impactful yoga class experiences — which is another desire I hear from the teachers that I mentor — then it is of great importance that you pursue and develop confidence in what and how you are teaching. As a yoga teacher, your ability to engage students in the practice and offer them an encounter with the practice that calls them back to their mat again and again is going to be less about your ability to creatively sequence or entertain students with asana tricks and more about your quiet, yet confident presence as teacher.

Students are smart. I also believe that confidence and trust are connected. When the students trust you, they will engage and respond. They will go where you lead them. This then raises the question — where are you leading students? And do you really trust in the teachings of yoga to get them there?

## Quiet Confidence

Confidence isn't loud or flashy. Within quiet confidence comes the belief of fully knowing, while believing, in what you are teaching. Within this quiet confidence, it's about the teachings of yoga and less about the teacher. The practice and teachings of yoga are bigger than we are as students and as teachers. This is an area where we get muddied in our understanding of our role, and we might take on the persona, or pursuit, toward teaching where we feel we must be on an ongoing quest to know more to present ourselves with credibility as if we needed to validate the teachings of yoga. From my experience, great freedom comes within the realization that, as a teacher, I am not the teachings. I say this because the lack of confidence you feel could quite possibly be coming from how you have identified with your role as teacher.

## Why Confidence Matters

If confidence can be recognized and the lack of confidence is an obstacle for yoga teachers, then let's explore how to move forward in developing confidence when it feels lacking. First, confidence amplifies quality and success. Confidence, or the lack of it, may be an obstacle, yet it's not the ultimate end result nor should it ever compensate for working toward a goal. Confidence is not a substitute for the quality and depth of your character. Even the most confident people need to feel confident in something — themselves, their work, or the activities and pursuits they identify with. Confidence alone will not stand — not for very long. Confidence must be coupled with contentment.

Perhaps, if you struggle with overcoming the obstacle of insecurity, then there is a need also to spend time reflecting upon where you are in your level of contentment. Are there areas where you feel disconnected? Is the feeling of insecurity really connected to an area of discontentment? This is a point of inquiry to spend some time reflecting upon so that you can ultimately clear the hurdle that equates to a lack of confidence.

Next, seek to better understand the source of your insecurity or discontentment so that you can come to know that true confidence is an essential part of the development of your character and the work you pursue as a teacher. Confidence can be conceptual and generalized, so this is where I want to highlight the word "true." You can be confident in general. True confidence acts as fuel on the fire of whatever we touch. This internal work will always need to be fueled to keep the fire going. Without the fuel, your fire will struggle to grow.

Thirdly, confidence is essential to your leadership and influence. What we do is a matter of technical skill. How we do it is a function of confidence. Here's where a balanced approach in your skill set comes in again. Relying solely on your technical skill set as a teacher is not going to be enough. Accumulating more trainings and even diving into the deeper study of a three-hundred-hour YTT before you're prepared and ready in a quest to accumulate more knowledge will not magically make you more confident. This consumption is not the sole key to teaching confidently. In fact, this approach could backfire and leave you feeling overwhelmed and even less confident.

Fourth, confidence isn't superficial. Being confident is about having substance. Confidence is not a byproduct of how much you know or how many credentials you've accumulated. If you are accumulating training after training but find you aren't actually applying the content of knowledge that you've been given, then you have become a collector. If this evaluation isn't made, then you will quickly become more confused and less focused on your unique purpose and calling as a teacher. As you are swept up in this pursuit, you might find yourself confused and lacking clear direction.

Lastly, when it comes to the importance of confidence, it is protection. Confidence manifests in a variety of ways. If we reside within the state of insecurity, we will wear this as a badge, and it will ultimately dictate the interactions we will have with others and how they interact with us. Confidence has a collective impact. In addition to enhancing our work and character, confidence also helps to protect us, physically and emotionally. Fundamentally, when we work on the development of confidence, we can better understand who we are, how we present ourselves in the world, and how the world will interact with us in return.

If you truly desire to engage and make meaningful connections with the students you lead, then it is important that you work on the relational development of confidence and presence as a teacher. It will support your ability to curate the type of relationship and interactions you desire, set healthy boundaries, and determine the impact you'll make in your community as a leader by teaching yoga.

## Reflective Exercise

Journal on the prompt of what you feel is your purpose for teaching yoga? What impact do you desire to make by teaching? Consider the intention behind what you write and evaluate the impact you make serving and connecting with others through the practice of yoga.

# Called to Teach Yoga

---

"Without service, we would not have a strong quality
of life. It's important to the person who serves
as well as the recipient. It's the way in which we
ourselves grow and develop."

– DOROTHY HEIGHT

In this lesson, explore how teaching yoga is a calling. It is a call from the heart to support and equip others within a practice designed to embrace a fuller experience of the sweetness of life. This worthy endeavor will require patience, endurance, and a deep understanding of who you are, as an individual and as a teacher. The calling to teach will invite you to use your unique gifts to teach others within a skillful and nurturing experience called a yoga class. It begins in the heart, and from the heart, you will lead with defined character and quiet confidence.

When I entered into my two-hundred-hour yoga teacher training with Rolf Gates, I had already been teaching yoga for eight years. What prompted me to embark on that journey under Rolf's guidance was this deep desire to expand and grow even more as a yoga teacher. I sensed and knew there was so much more. I would then go on to complete my three-hundred-hour training with Rolf shortly after the completion of that two-hundred-hour experience.

During that first weekend, Rolf shared his journey with us, his calling to teach, and his calling to become a teacher of teachers. I sat there inspired, and in that moment, I, too, felt the calling to not only continue to teach others but to pursue and become a teacher of teachers myself. The yoga practice has been a gift to me, and I have committed to the pursuit and quest to learn, grow, and study so that I might be better equipped and ready to give that gift to others and to motivate and inspire yoga teachers in their pursuit to teach. To me, this is the calling to be a yoga teacher. To give freely of that which has been given. For me, it is to give from the place within me where I forged the gap many years ago when my mom passed and I stood wondering what I would do that felt fulfilling or of service as it had felt to serve and take care of my mother in the last days of her life. That day as I stood in my teacher training experience, I knew the gift had been given to me, in turn. It was time for me to give it to others.

The path of teaching has not been easy, and I would never try to convince you otherwise. It requires work. It requires patience and endurance. It has been a journey like none other and has granted me many beautiful moments to connect with others along the way. I am grateful for each teaching opportunity that I have had and the ones that are yet to come. I am grateful to the teachers who have come before me, the ones who have poured themselves into me and seen within me the teacher who has always resided there. It is my hope and desire that this book has supported you in the same way. Teaching yoga is truly a most worthy endeavor, and I wish you well along life's journey and along the pathway of service as you develop and grow as a yoga teacher.

## Reflective Exercise

List the qualities of character and leadership that you possess as a teacher. Reflect on how you can use your gifts to share the practice with others. Now, where do you feel called to serve your community as a yoga teacher?

# Afterword

A call to excellence, a call for us all. A call for yoga teachers to teach from the heart.

---

"For out of the abundance of the heart the mouth speaks."

— JESUS, MATTHEW 12:34 ESV

Perhaps the call to teach yoga is a natural extension of who we are. The Yoga Sutras of Patanjali suggests that deep within us is a well of stillness. Over the past two decades, as a yoga practitioner and teacher, I have experienced this well, and from the depths of this well, I believe there is a wellspring that also comes forth from the depths of our hearts. A heart that desires to explore the vast terrain of a spiritual plane that reaches farther than our human comprehension and desire to meet that which is bigger than ourselves. For me, this terrain is where I encounter my Creator, God and Jesus.

Our character, confidence, and, ultimately, our leadership flows from the overflowing spring of our heart. A heart of service and connection emerges from the wellspring with a desire to encounter others and to share a moment in time, in the presence of that which is greater than we all are, sharing an experience, and the collective hope of the plight of humanity and the elimination of suffering. It's within these moments that we can experience a glimpse of this realization, and through the yoga practice we come to know our capacity to reside in this heart space with consistency. And once again, we return to joy and are hopeful.

From the calling to teach, we are then challenged to dig deep and are presented with the choice of teaching from this wholehearted wellspring deep within us. The call is to share and support others along their journeys so that collectively, we can encounter the stillness and peace and ultimately experience the fullness of human life and experience. It is my desire that through the lessons I have shared in this book, as a yoga teacher and ultimately as a child of God, that you will come to know the fullness of your path of teaching and sharing the practice of yoga with others. Use the lessons to support your development and refinement of character, confidence, and leadership within the spirit and heart of service and connection with others.

# About the Author

SANDY RAPER, E-RYT 500, RYS, YACEP, YOGA MEDICINE®
THERAPEUTIC SPECIALIST

Sandy Raper is an esteemed and devoted yoga teacher with an illustrious career spanning more than two decades. Her unwavering commitment to the field has positioned her as a fervent advocate for fellow yoga teachers. Throughout her career, she has played a pivotal role in the training, equipping, and mentoring of teachers on a global scale.

Sandy Raper's credentials and certifications are a testament to her extensive and diverse training background. Ranging from foundational certifications to advanced training in therapeutic applications, her expertise runs deep and reflects a profound understanding of the intricacies found within the practice of yoga.

Sandy's notable contributions lie in her active involvement in creating comprehensive course curricula for equipping and training yoga teachers, including at the college level. She has also been a featured presenter at educational conferences, including two appearances at the Yoga Medicine® Innovation Conference. Additionally, Sandy has offered various continuing education workshops and training sessions to further enhance and elevate the skills and knowledge of yoga teachers.

Beyond her accomplishments as an educator, Sandy Raper is deeply invested in the evolution of the yoga practice while seeking creative methods for teaching and sharing. She brings a unique perspective to the yoga community, blending tradition with contemporary insights. Sandy Raper is not only an expert in the theoretical aspects of yoga but also a practitioner committed to embodying the principles of the profound wholeness one can experience through the application of the practices of yoga.

Driven by a strong passion to inspire, encourage, and equip yoga teachers further, Sandy Raper took an accelerated step in 2020 by creating the Beyond Yoga Teacher Training Podcast and Mentorship Program. Beyond the yoga classroom, Sandy Raper resides in North Carolina, where she enjoys serving her community and local church, traveling, and spending time with her family and friends. She lives her yoga off the mat in balance as a wife, mother of three, and caretaker.

**Connect and learn more:** www.sandyraper.com
**IG:** sandyraperyoga
**FB:** Sandy Raper Yoga